JUICING FOR WELLNESS IN
YOUR NAMA®

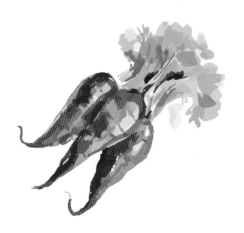

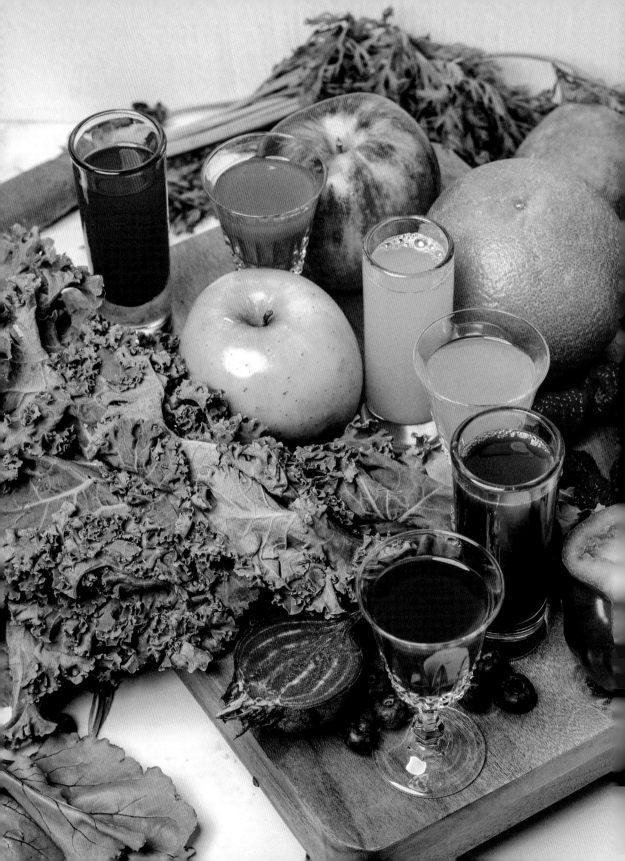

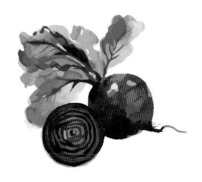

JUICING FOR WELLNESS IN
YOUR NAMA®

60 Healthy Recipes to
Easily Boost Your Nutritional Intake

JEANETTE VELASCO SHANE

Creator of Juicy Juicing J

PAGE STREET
PUBLISHING CO.

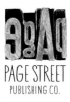

PAGE STREET
PUBLISHING CO.

First published in 2024 by
Page Street Publishing Co.
27 Congress Street, Suite 1511
Salem, MA 01970
www.pagestreetpublishing.com

Distributed by Macmillan, sales in Canada by The Canadian Manda Group.

28   27   26   25   24   1   2   3   4   5

ISBN-13: 979-8-89003-980-4

Library of Congress Control Number: 2023936751

Edited by Marissa Giambelluca
Cover and book design by Elena Van Horn for Page Street Publishing Co.
Photography by Jeremy Shane

Printed and bound in the United States of America

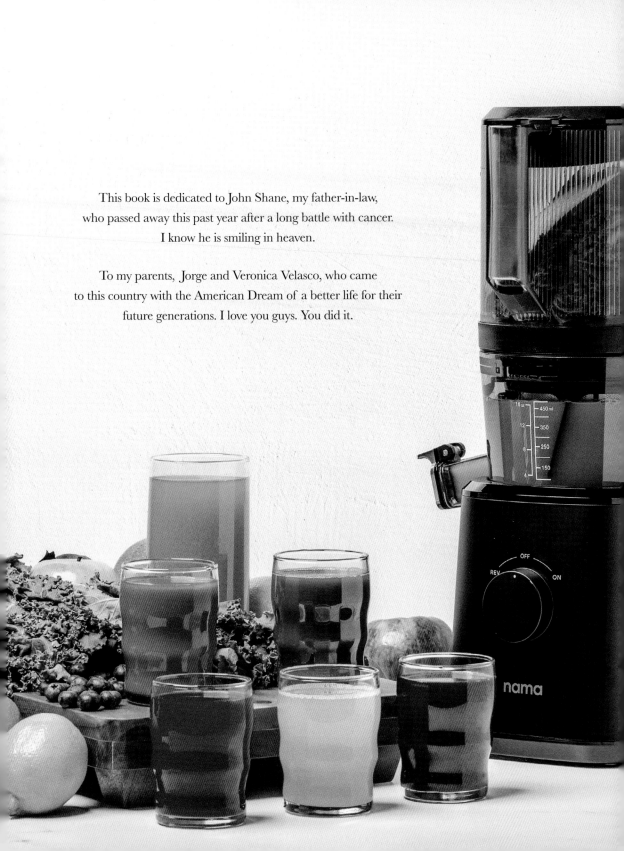

This book is dedicated to John Shane, my father-in-law,
who passed away this past year after a long battle with cancer.
I know he is smiling in heaven.

To my parents, Jorge and Veronica Velasco, who came
to this country with the American Dream of a better life for their
future generations. I love you guys. You did it.

CONTENTS

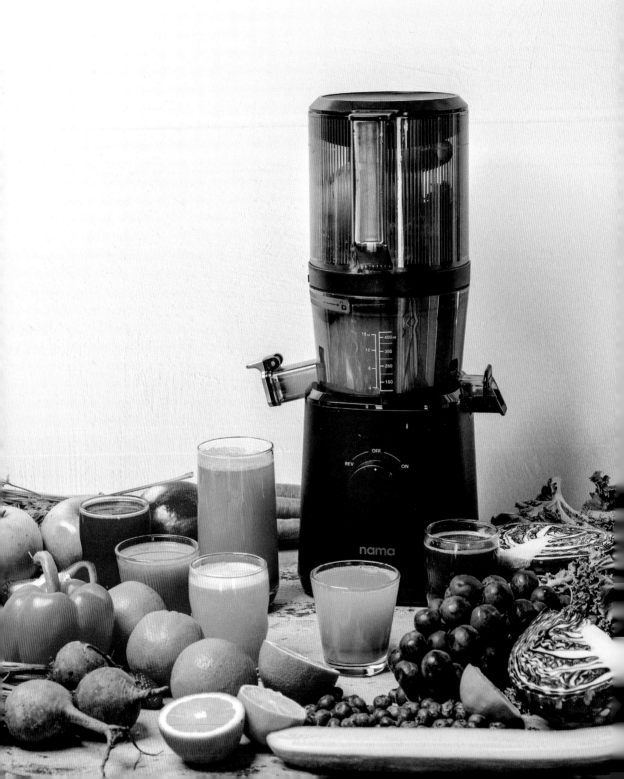

INTRODUCTION

Hi! I'm so glad you're here. If you told me a year ago I would write my own juice recipe book, I would not have believed it. I feel incredibly blessed to have this amazing community and the opportunity to share what I love. I started posting my juicing recipes because I saw a need for a space where seasoned juicers and newbies could come to find simple recipes no matter what their juice journey looked like.

I wanted my recipes to be beautiful, helpful, inviting and, of course, delicious and packed with nutrients. I wanted to show that juicing isn't something unattainable— anyone can do it. Whether you're vegan, vegetarian, plant-based or simply looking to get more fruits and veggies in your day-to-day life, you are in the right place.

My juicing journey began at a young age. My mom had a health scare that changed a lot of what we consumed on a day-to-day basis when I was growing up. We used food as medicine and used juices to help maintain our health. Being Mexican, my mom was familiar with a lot of home remedies and used ingredients to treat various ailments, such as beets for iron, carrots to help vision and bananas for cramps. You name it, she had a remedy.

My mom laid a lot of the foundation I have now when it comes to juicing and health and wellness. I struggled with being borderline anemic in my teenage years, and my mom was always making me an apple-beet-carrot juice (what everyone calls an ABC juice) when she noticed me getting sluggish and tired during the day. I am a high-energy person so it was definitely noticeable when I needed some iron. She also had juices ready for me when I had a cross-country meet or an active day ahead. Thanks to my mom and juicing, I was able to maintain my health and get the nutrients my body needed.

I stopped juicing when I got to college. After I graduated and went into the corporate world, I started to realize how much I missed it. I wanted the energy I felt when I was drinking juices. It took the pandemic to make my way back into juicing and, well, here we are today.

I drink a juice a day, sometimes two. This routine helps me feel energized and has so many positive effects on my body. I have glowing skin, healthy hair and nails, improved digestion and better workouts. I rarely have headaches or get sick. I feel better now than I did in college, and I look forward to my juice every day. Juicing isn't a diet. It's a lifestyle that I hope will be passed down to future generations.

Drinking the rainbow is a great way to make sure our bodies are getting what they need every day. Each color group has its own set of superfood powers. That's why this book contains recipes in the colors of the rainbow. Fruits and veggies are powerful, and juicing is a great way to add them to your diet. Once you see the benefits and changes in your body, it will be hard to stop.

No matter where you are starting from, I'm glad you're here. I want this book to help keep you motivated, consistent and excited about your juicing journey. I hope that the recipes bring energy, health and wellness into your life—just like they have in mine.

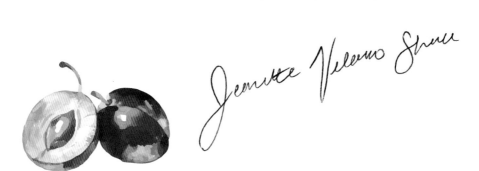

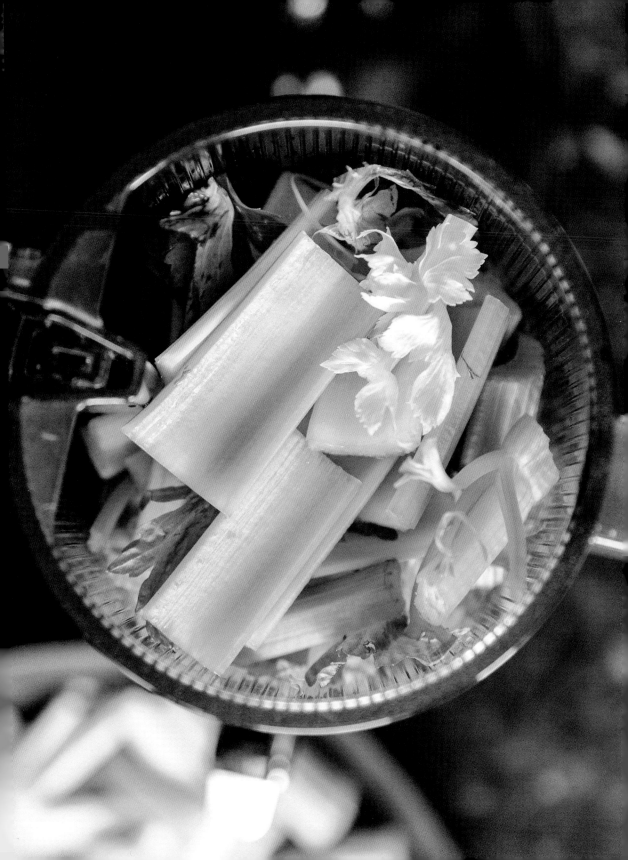

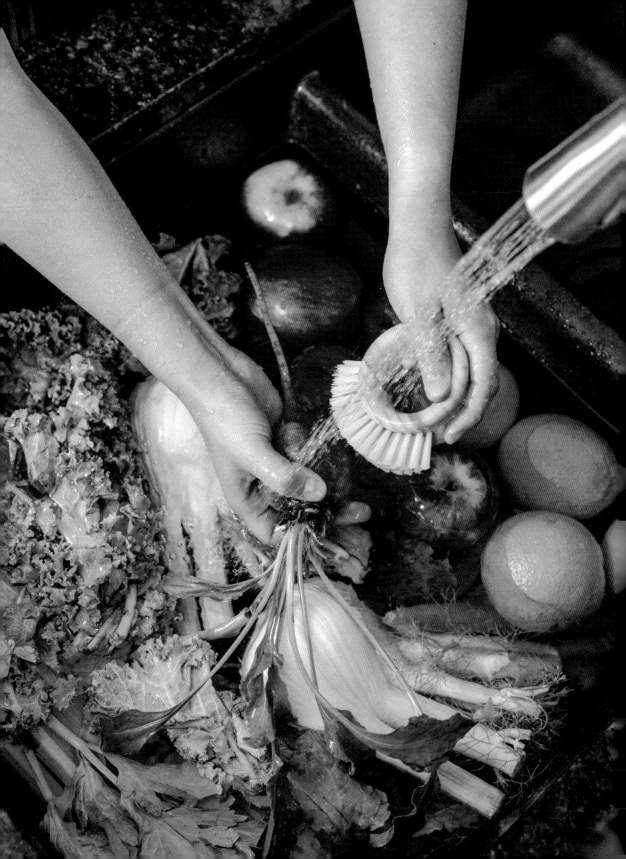

Why I Chose Nama

I knew I wanted a cold press juicer. Cold press juicers maximize the amount of juice that is extracted from produce. They also minimize oxidation to preserve nutrients, vitamins and phytonutrients. After six months of researching, reading reviews and watching reviews, the Nama juicer was the best fit for me and my lifestyle. It has a clean, beautiful, easy-to-use design, and I love what they represent as a company. I wanted to maximize the amount of juice I was getting from my produce, and I love seeing how dry the pulp is when I juice. It saves me time (e.g., less cutting, hands-free). It's also quiet compared to many juicers, and I'm not worried I'll wake up everyone in our building when I juice.

Tips to Optimize Your Nama Juicing Experience

- Assemble the chamber set first, then add it to the base. (Don't assemble it on the base; it won't turn on.)

- Wash your juicer right after you use it. It's faster, and this will help reduce staining.

- Layer your ingredients with leafy greens and soft fruits/veggies at the bottom and hard fruits/veggies on top. This helps create a natural pressure for a smoother juicing process.

- Cut more fibrous produce, such as celery, pineapple, kale and spinach, into smaller pieces. This allows your produce to flow through the juicer effectively, especially if you are loading a bigger batch.

How to Wash Fruits and Veggies

I like to wash my produce in vinegar, water and baking soda. Mix one part vinegar to three parts cold water in a large bowl, leaving room for your fruit and veggies. Add your ingredients to the bowl, and sprinkle them with baking soda. Give it all a stir with your hands, and let it sit for about five minutes. Use your veggie and fruit brush, and scrub!

I also often find myself reaching for a premade veggie wash because it's a quicker method. My favorite veggie wash cleaner, Rebel Green®, is specifically labeled as great for juicing. Once you've washed your produce, rinse it and you are ready to start juicing.

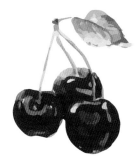

How to Store Juices

It's best to maximize the amount of nutrients you are consuming, so drinking your juice fresh is ideal. But making fresh juice every day may not be realistic, especially if you have school, work, sports, kids' activities and more!

When stored properly, cold-pressed juices last up to 72 hours nutrient-wise in the fridge. I love to use glass mason jars to store my juices. If you choose to use plastic, be aware that it can alter the taste and may leach into your juices.

Fill your container all the way to the top to minimize oxidation of your juice. The more air in your container, the faster the juice will oxidize. A lot of my juice recipes have optional lime or lemon. Adding citrus fruit will help prevent oxidation. And remember, juice does settle when stored in the fridge. Make sure you give it a good shake before drinking.

If you don't plan on drinking your juice within 72 hours, freeze it to preserve the juice's nutrients. The flavor of your juice doesn't change after freezing in mason jars! The batch juicing chapter (page 87) has more details on how to freeze your juices.

Ways to Use Pulp

When you've finished juicing, don't throw out your pulp! Pulp has tons of nutrients, and you can maximize the use for it. Here are a few ideas:

- **Overnight oats:** Add one part pulp to two parts oats to a mason jar. Fill it with your favorite plant-based milk, and place it in your fridge overnight for a ready-made breakfast treat.

- **Baked goods:** Add about ¼ to ½ cup (weight varies) of pulp to your favorite baked goods recipe.

- **Freeze for smoothies:** Add the pulp to ice cube trays along with a little bit of water to help it freeze. Freeze, then pop a cube or two into smoothies for added flavor and nutrition.

- **Veggie broth:** Add about ¼ cup (weight varies) of pulp to ½ cup (120 ml) of your broth. Veggie pulp works best for this.

- **Eat it like a salad:** Add the pulp to a bowl with your favorite salad dressing and enjoy.

- **Composting:** Add it as compost to your garden.

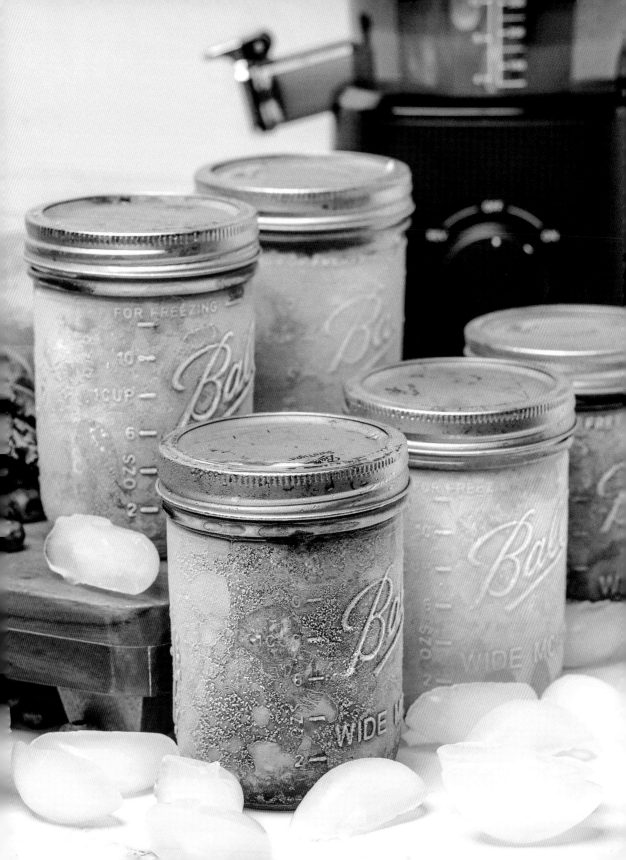

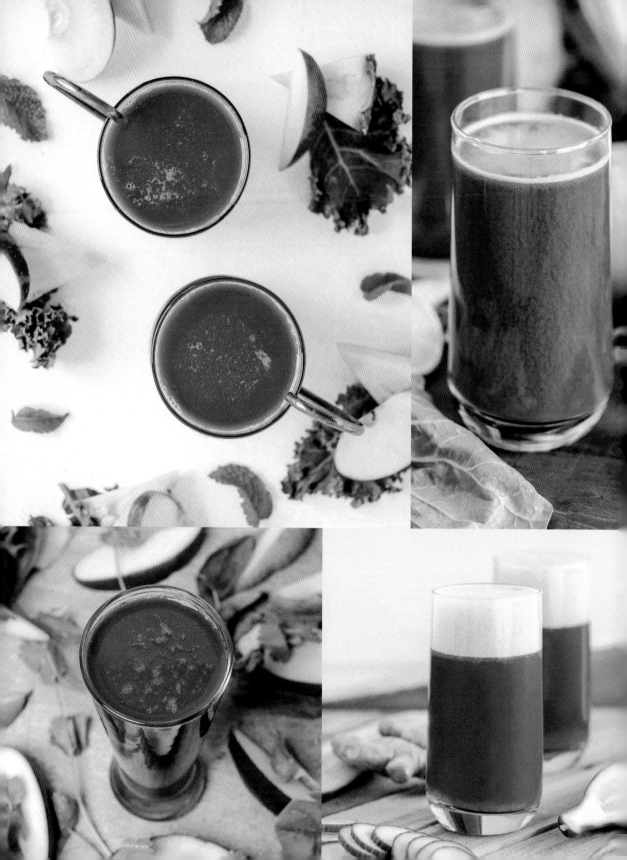

GET YOUR GREENS
GREEN JUICES

Add more veggies into your life! Some people love leafy greens, and others hate them. Either way, many people struggle to get enough greens in their diet. I get it. It was a challenge for me. I don't mind greens, but I didn't look forward to eating them or go out of my way to eat them.

Juicing has made it so simple—and delicious—to get my daily greens in. And drinking your greens is a great way to nourish your body. Green fruits and veggies contain many essential nutrients, such as phytonutrients, folate, vitamin K, magnesium, antioxidants and more. They also have anti-inflammatory properties, support the immune system, promote gut and heart health and support your body in fighting chronic illness and cancer cells.

I created these green juices that I am sure you and your whole family will love. They'll help you get all the green goodness every day!

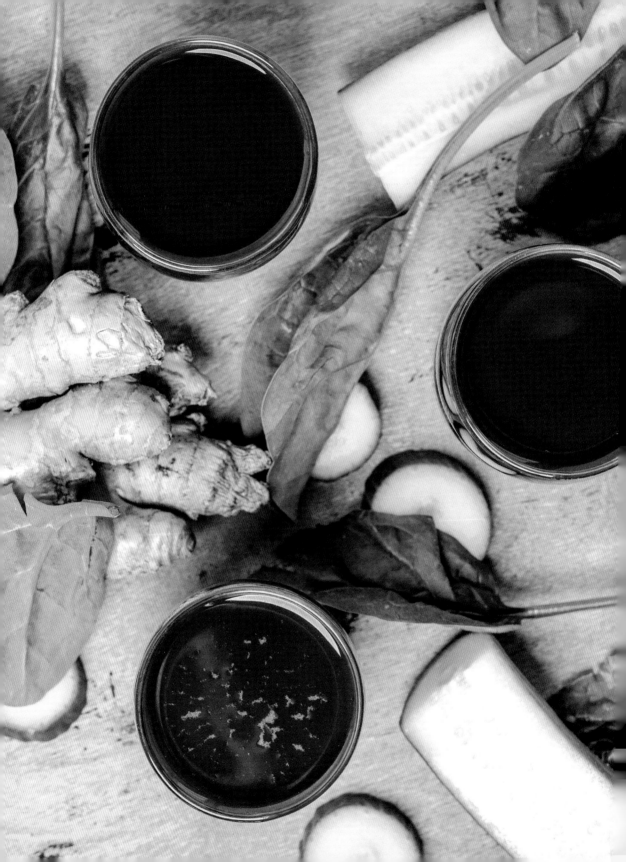

SIMPLY VERDE

This simple juice is full of leafy green goodness. It has nutrients that support healthy skin, hair, bone health and more. It's simple to make with easy-to-find grocery store ingredients. This veggie-packed juice is super smooth and hydrating, and it will leave you feeling refreshed and energized.

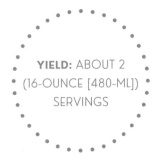

YIELD: ABOUT 2 (16-OUNCE [480-ML]) SERVINGS

GET JUICING!

Wash your leafy greens and other produce, and get ready to prep.

Cut the romaine leaves in half. Cut the cucumber into quarters to fit easily in the hopper. I like to peel my ginger with a potato peeler, but you can leave it unpeeled if you prefer. Cut the ginger into smaller pieces for a smoother juicing process.

Add the ingredients to the hopper in this order: First layer your leafy greens, then add the cucumber and ginger.

Once it's loaded, turn on the juicer and run it until all the ingredients are juiced.

JUICING LINE UP

4 PACKED CUPS (140 G) SPINACH

2 ROMAINE HEARTS

1 ENGLISH CUCUMBER

1 (3-INCH [7.5-CM]) PIECE OF GINGER

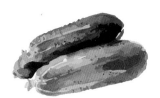

NOTES

- I prefer to use English cucumbers for juices. They have a fresher, sweeter taste to them.
- If you can't find romaine hearts, you can use one head of romaine lettuce instead.

POWER UP

This juice is a great way to boost your morning!

I grew up with people telling me to eat my spinach to make me big and strong. This incredible combination of leafy greens, sweet pears and cooling cucumbers supports healthy hair and skin, provides essential nutrients and vitamins and supports your body with powerful antioxidants!

• •

GET JUICING!

Wash your leafy greens and other produce, and get ready to prep.

Remove the stems from the pears. Cut the cucumber into quarters to fit easily in the hopper.

Add the ingredients to the hopper in this order: First layer your leafy greens, then add the pears and cucumber on top for a smoother juicing process.

Once it's loaded, turn on the juicer and run it until all the ingredients are juiced.

• •

NOTE: Kale is more fibrous. Feel free to chop it for a smoother juicing process.

YIELD: ABOUT 2 (16-OUNCE [480-ML]) SERVINGS

JUICING LINE UP

6 PACKED CUPS (210 G) SPINACH

6 PACKED CUPS (480 G) KALE

2 PEARS

1 ENGLISH CUCUMBER

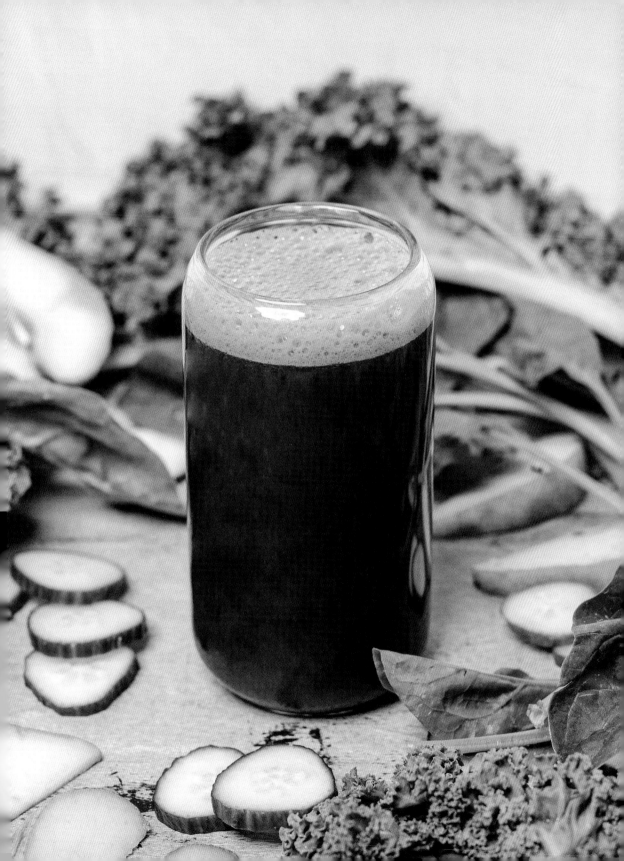

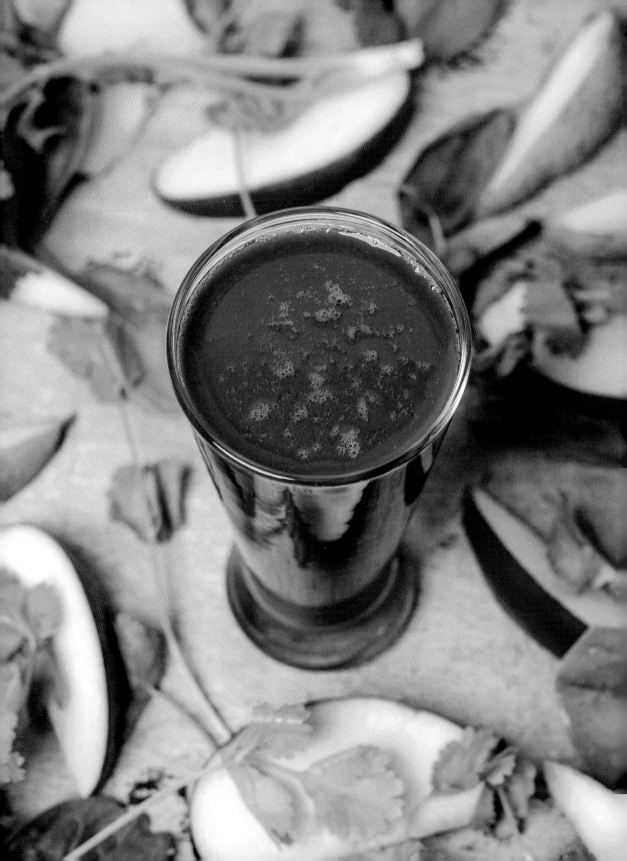

KICKING GREENS

I love cilantro. It adds incredible flavor to so many of my favorite Mexican dishes! What surprised me is how much I like it in my juice. Cilantro in juice? Trust me; this is one you want to try. It's bold, smooth and delicious and adds just the right amount of sweet kick to your juice. If you're new to green juices, this is a great one to ease you into more of the veggie-heavy juices. These fruits and veggies are known to support the body's natural detoxification, brain health, immune system and digestive health.

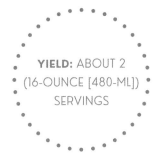

YIELD: ABOUT 2 (16-OUNCE [480-ML]) SERVINGS

GET JUICING!

Wash your leafy greens and other produce, and get ready to prep.

Remove any wilted or slimy leaves from the cilantro and spinach. Use a knife to remove the peel from the limes. Remove the stems from the pears.

There is no need to peel the apples, but you can core them. Nama suggests coring because apple seeds are known to have toxicity; I prefer to core my apples for juicing.

Add the ingredients to the hopper in this order: First layer your leafy greens, then add the limes, pears and apple on top for a smoother juicing process.

Once it's loaded, turn on the juicer and run it until all the ingredients are juiced.

JUICING LINE UP

½ CUP (20 G) CILANTRO

8 PACKED CUPS (280 G) SPINACH

2 LIMES

2 PEARS

1 APPLE

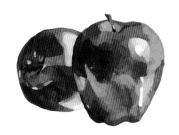

NOTE: Trim the ends of your cilantro and spinach if they have become brown and a little wilted, as this can affect the taste.

ELECTRIC COOLER

This juice is packed with vitamin C, antioxidants and anti-inflammatory properties. This combo is sweet, tart and electric. It will have you saying WOAH as soon as you take the first sip—just ask my husband. It's great for kids, and it's a great way to add in a veggie they might not try on its own, like bok choy. Think of it as a delicious, immune system–boosting green punch that you'll want to share with all your friends!

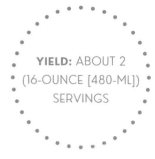

YIELD: ABOUT 2 (16-OUNCE [480-ML]) SERVINGS

GET JUICING!

Wash your leafy greens and other produce, and get ready to prep.

Use a knife to remove the peel from the lime. Chop the bok choy into smaller pieces to fit in the hopper. Remove the crown from the pineapple and remove the skin. I don't core my pineapple; I like to keep it because there are many nutrients found in the core. Once you remove the skin from your pineapple, cut it into small chunks.

There is no need to peel the apple, but you can core it. Nama suggests coring because apple seeds are known to have toxicity; I prefer to core my apples when juicing.

Add the ingredients to the hopper in this order: First layer your kale, then add the lime, bok choy, pineapple and apple on top for a smoother juicing process.

Once it's loaded, turn on the juicer and run it until all the ingredients are juiced.

JUICING LINE UP

12 KALE LEAVES

1 LIME

6 BOK CHOY LEAVES

½ OF A PINEAPPLE

1 GRANNY SMITH APPLE

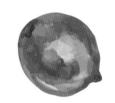

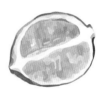

TIP: Chop the leafy greens into smaller pieces for a smoother juicing process.

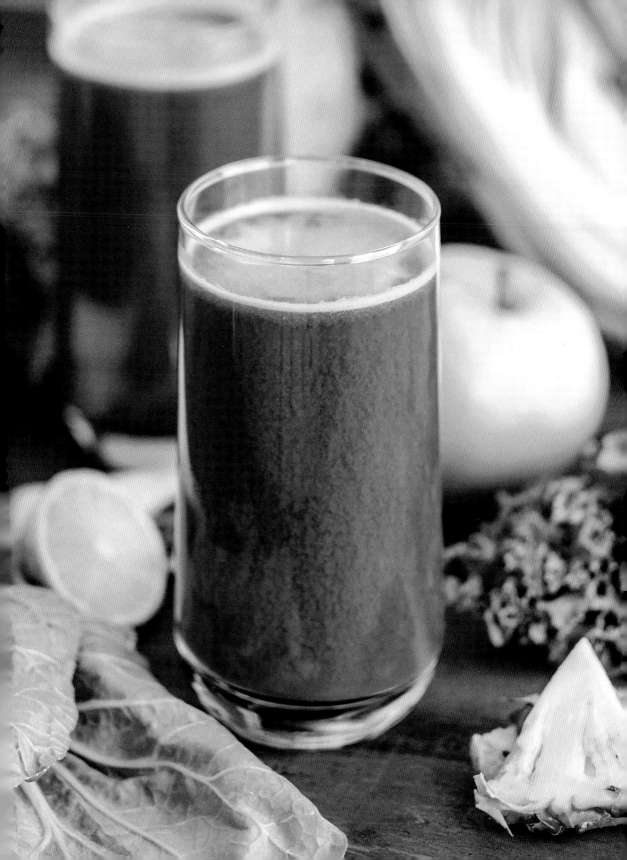

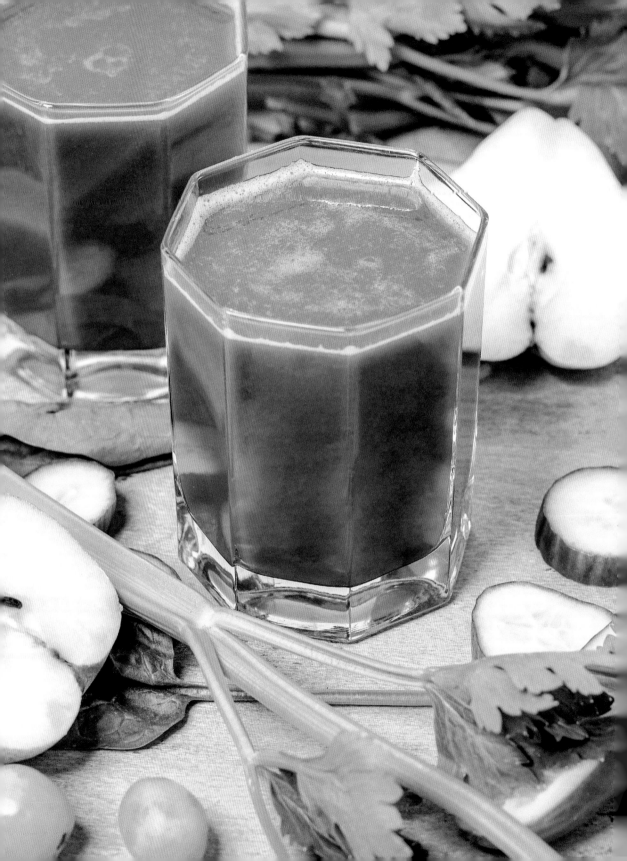

SMOOTH COOL CUE

Feel cool as a cucumber with this smooth, hydrating juice. If you're looking for a juice on the sweeter side, this is the one for you. This combo is packed with antioxidants and helps support healthy skin, eye health and more. If you're new to green juices, this is a great one to start with!

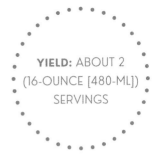

YIELD: ABOUT 2 (16-OUNCE [480-ML]) SERVINGS

GET JUICING!

Wash your leafy greens and other produce, and get ready to prep.

Remove the stems from the grapes and pears. Cut the celery ribs into quarters for a smoother juicing process. Cut the cucumbers into quarters to fit easily in the hopper.

Add the ingredients to the hopper in this order: First layer your spinach, grapes, celery and pears, then add the cucumbers on top for a smoother juicing process.

Once it's loaded, turn on the juicer and run it until all the ingredients are juiced.

JUICING LINE UP

2 PACKED CUPS (70 G) SPINACH

2 CUPS TABLE GRAPES (66 GRAPES)

2 RIBS CELERY

2 PEARS

2 ENGLISH CUCUMBERS

NOTE: I prefer to use English cucumbers. The flavor tastes better in my opinion.

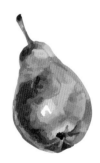

RADIANT GREENS

If you want to focus on your complexion, this Radiant Greens juice is the way to go. Switch up your typical leafy greens with Swiss chard. It's an easy leafy green to juice, and it isn't as fibrous as spinach and kale. Plus, it helps support your bone health!

YIELD: ABOUT 2 (16-OUNCE [480-ML]) SERVINGS

GET JUICING!

Wash your leafy greens and other produce, and get ready to prep.

Cut the cucumbers into quarters to fit easily in the hopper. I like to peel my ginger with a potato peeler, but you can leave it unpeeled if you prefer. Cut the ginger into smaller pieces for a smoother juicing process.

There is no need to peel the apples, but you can core them. Nama suggests coring because apple seeds are known to have toxicity; I prefer to core my apples when juicing.

Add the ingredients to the hopper in this order: First layer your chard, then add the cucumbers, ginger and apples on top for a smoother juicing process.

Once it's loaded, turn on the juicer and run it until all the ingredients are juiced.

JUICING LINE UP

12 SWISS CHARD LEAVES

2 ENGLISH CUCUMBERS

1 (3-INCH [7.5-CM]) PIECE OF GINGER

2 GRANNY SMITH APPLES

NOTE: Granny Smith apples give this one a nice tart flavor.

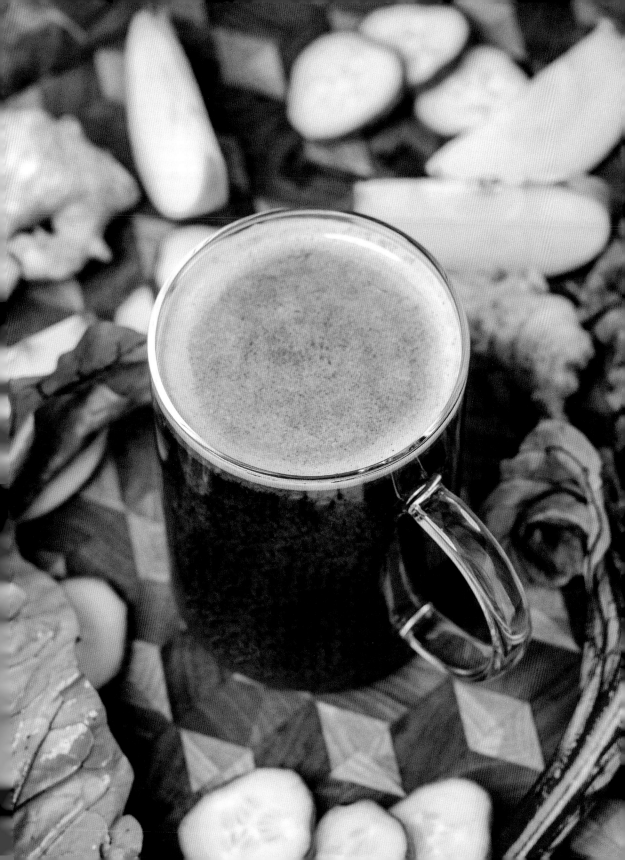

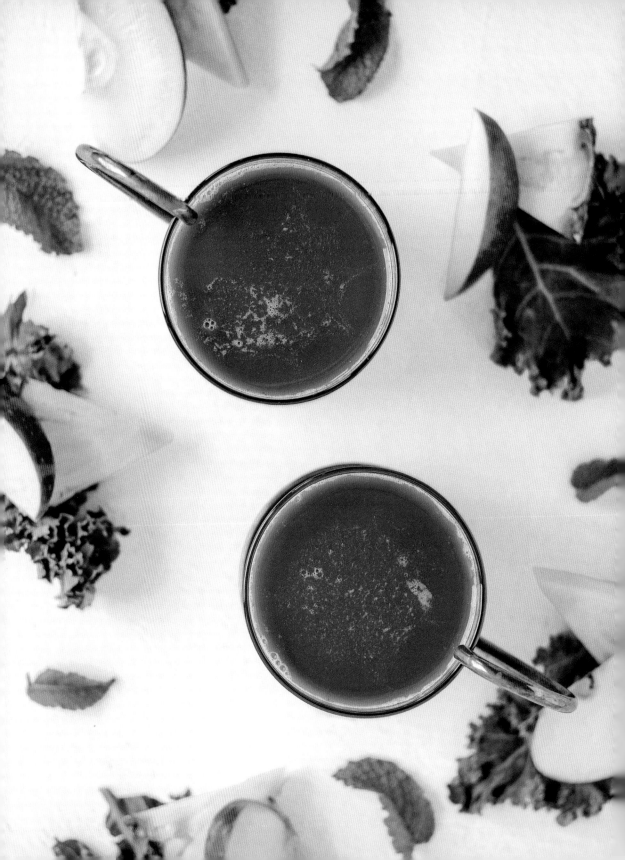

THE WORKS

This drink is inspired by one of my favorite drinks to get at a juice bar when I'm traveling—with more greens added to this version. The fruit and leafy greens are a powerful, natural way to reduce bloating and support bone health. Save your money and make this at home. And for that true juice bar experience, pour it over ice and sip away.

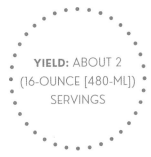

YIELD: ABOUT 2 (16-OUNCE [480-ML]) SERVINGS

· ·

GET JUICING!

Wash your leafy greens and other produce, and get ready to prep.

Remove the crown from the pineapple and remove the skin. I don't core my pineapple; I like to keep it because there are many nutrients found in the core. Once you remove the skin from your pineapple, cut it into small chunks.

There is no need to peel the apples, but you can core them. Nama suggests coring because apple seeds are known to have toxicity; I prefer to core my apples when juicing.

Add the ingredients to the hopper in this order: First layer your leafy greens, then add the pineapple and apples on top for a smoother juicing process.

Once it's loaded, turn on the juicer and run it until all the ingredients are juiced.

JUICING LINE UP

4 PACKED CUPS (320 G) KALE

12 MINT LEAVES

½ OF A PINEAPPLE

2 PINK LADY® APPLES

· ·

NOTES

- Kale is more fibrous, so feel free to chop it for a smoother juicing process.
- You can use different apples for this; Cosmic Crisp® and Honeycrisp are great alternatives!

MORNING GREEN BOOST

Support your body's natural detoxification! Bok choy is known to have anticancer properties, and it supports your gut health and bone health. This juice will have you feeling good and ready to take on the day.

YIELD: ABOUT 2 (16-OUNCE [480-ML]) SERVINGS

. . . .

GET JUICING!

Wash your leafy greens and other produce, and get ready to prep.

Peel the lemon and cut it in half. Remove the stems from the pears. Chop the bok choy into smaller pieces to fit in the hopper. Cut the celery ribs into quarters for a smoother juicing process.

Add the ingredients to the hopper in this order: First layer your kale, then add the lemon, pears, bok choy and celery on top for a smoother juicing process.

Once it's loaded, turn on the juicer and run it until all the ingredients are juiced.

JUICING LINE UP

10 KALE LEAVES

1 LEMON

2 PEARS

6 BOK CHOY LEAVES

8 RIBS CELERY

. . . .

NOTE: Adding lemon helps enhance this juice by adding flavor. It also helps to keep it nice and fresh if you plan on drinking it the next day.

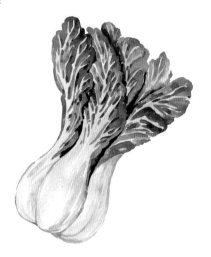

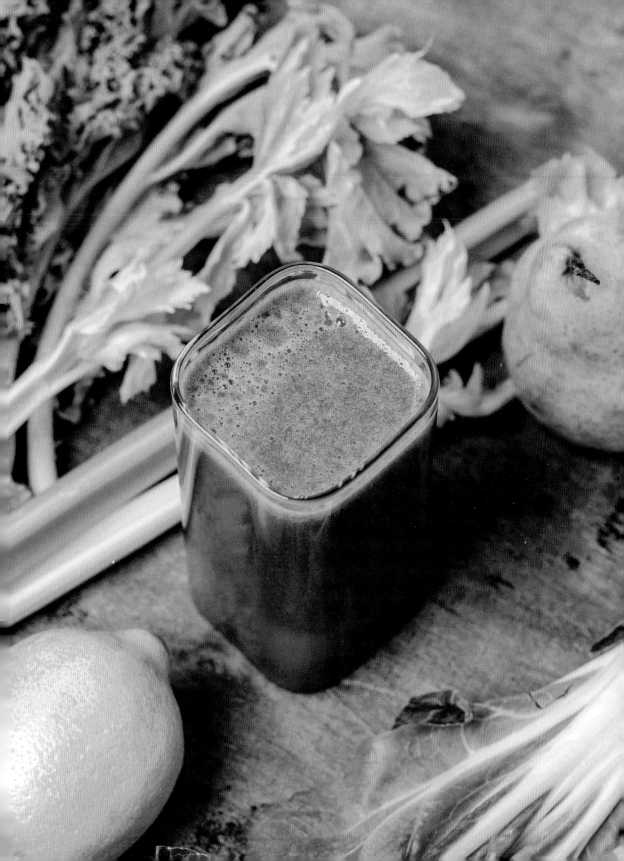

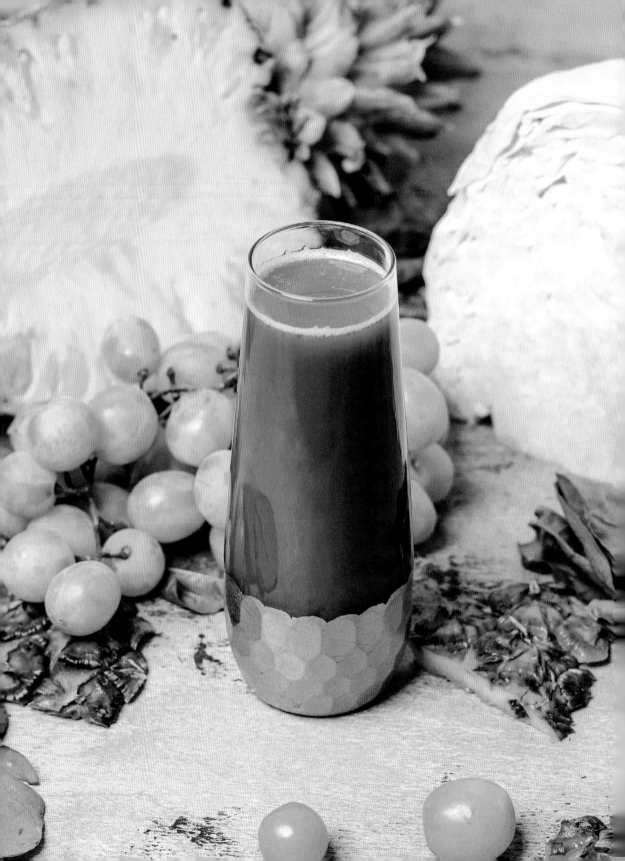

SUPER GS

Get ready for sweetness and a whole lot of gut-supporting goodness. Green cabbage has a milder taste compared to purple cabbage. It also has similar properties, such as fighting inflammation, being antioxidant-rich and improving digestion. Green cabbage is not a veggie I usually eat on its own, so being able to get its health benefits in this juice is a win-win for me!

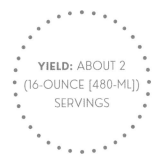

YIELD: ABOUT 2 (16-OUNCE [480-ML]) SERVINGS

GET JUICING!

Wash your leafy greens and other produce, and get ready to prep.

Remove the stems from the grapes. Remove the crown from the pineapple and remove the skin. I don't core my pineapple; I like to keep it because there are many nutrients found in the core. Once you remove the skin from your pineapple, cut it into small chunks.

Remove a few of the outer leaves from the cabbage, including any that are damaged or wilted. Cut it into pieces to fit easily in the hopper.

Add the ingredients to the hopper in this order: First layer your spinach, then add the grapes, pineapple and cabbage on top for a smoother juicing process.

Once it's loaded, turn on the juicer and run it until all the ingredients are juiced.

TIP: For easier washing, cut cabbages in half. I spray them with a veggie wash (page 13), then rinse them.

JUICING LINE UP

6 PACKED CUPS (210 G) SPINACH

1½ CUPS GREEN GRAPES (40 SMALL)

½ OF A PINEAPPLE

½ OF A CABBAGE

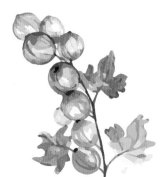

JUMP-START

Feeling bloated? Having digestive issues? Don't sweat it. Try this juice combo! Fennel gives this juice a mild anise flavor, and it is known to help aid digestion and have anti-inflammatory properties. If you're feeling sluggish in the morning, the taste of fennel in this juice will be sure to give you the start you need for the day.

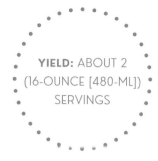

YIELD: ABOUT 2 (16-OUNCE [480-ML]) SERVINGS

. . . .

GET JUICING!

Wash all your produce and get ready to prep.

Chop the fennel into smaller chunks to fit into the juicer. Remove the stems from the pears. Cut the cucumbers into quarters to fit easily in the hopper.

Add the ingredients to the hopper in this order: First layer your fennel, then add the pears and cucumbers on top for a smoother juicing process.

Once it's loaded, turn on the juicer and run it until all the ingredients are juiced.

JUICING LINE UP

2 FENNEL BULBS

2 PEARS

2 ENGLISH CUCUMBERS

. . . .

TIP: Juice the fennel leaves if they are still attached. They add extra nutrition and more flavor and reduce waste.

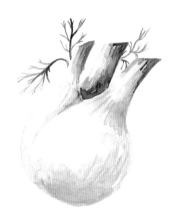

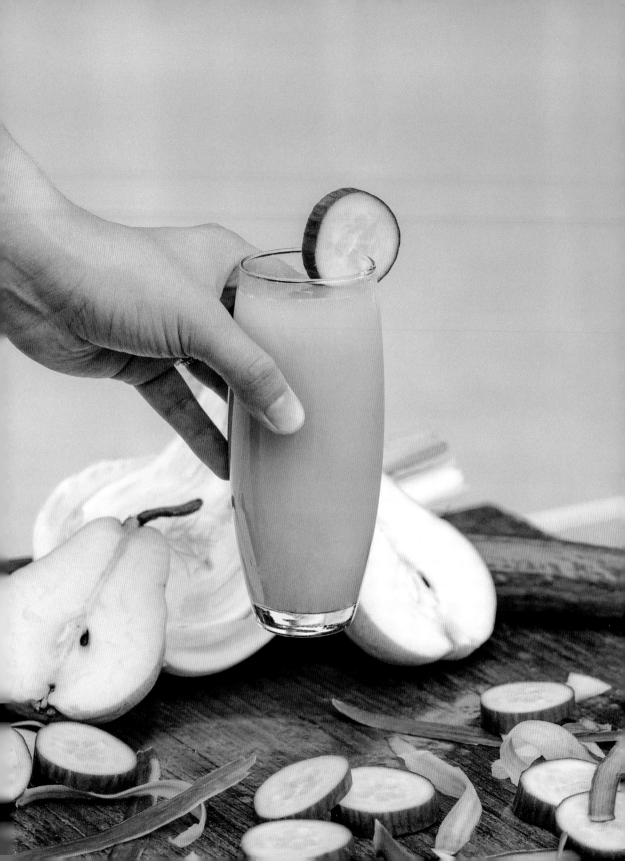

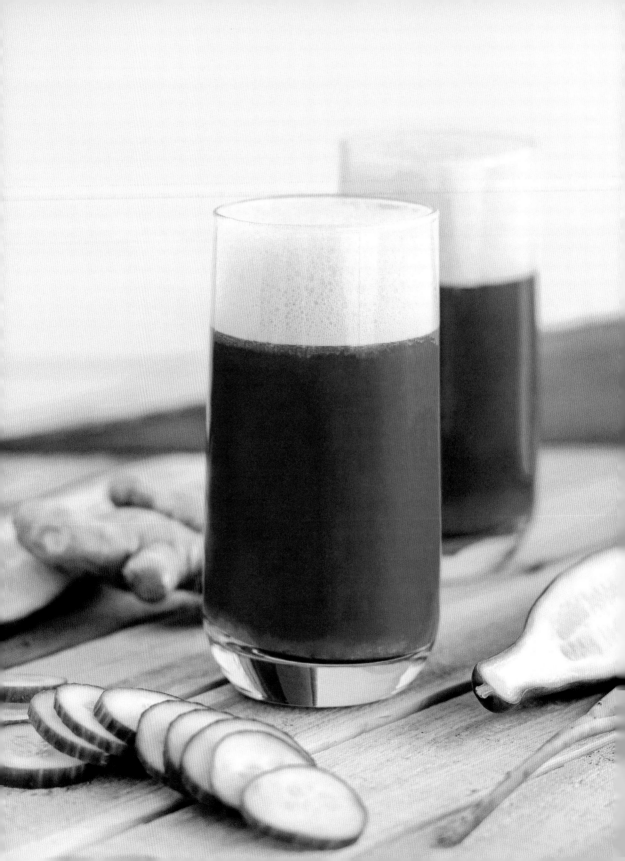

CALMING CUCUMBER

Glowing skin starts from the inside. This is one of my favorite juices. Aloe is great at supporting your digestive system; colon health; healthy, glowing skin and more! This juice is incredibly simple, plus it's soothing to the stomach and helps with bloating. It is a great natural remedy if you are experiencing an upset stomach.

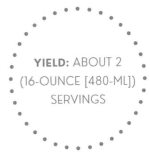

YIELD: ABOUT 2 (16-OUNCE [480-ML]) SERVINGS

GET JUICING!

Wash all your produce and get ready to prep.

Cut the cucumbers into quarters to fit easily in the hopper. I like to peel my ginger with a potato peeler, but you can leave it unpeeled if you prefer. Cut the ginger into smaller pieces for a smoother juicing process.

Add the ingredients to the hopper in this order: First layer your aloe, then add the cucumbers and ginger on top for a smoother juicing process.

Once it's loaded, turn on the juicer and run it until all the ingredients are juiced.

JUICING LINE UP

2 CUPS (480 ML) ALOE GEL

5 ENGLISH CUCUMBERS

2 (3-INCH [7.5-CM]) PIECES OF GINGER

TIPS

- If you are using aloe from the plant, you can run aloe pulp through the juicer again. Save a cucumber until the end so it can help push the pulp through the juicer.
- Aloe does foam; don't remove foam from the juice—aloe is in it as well.

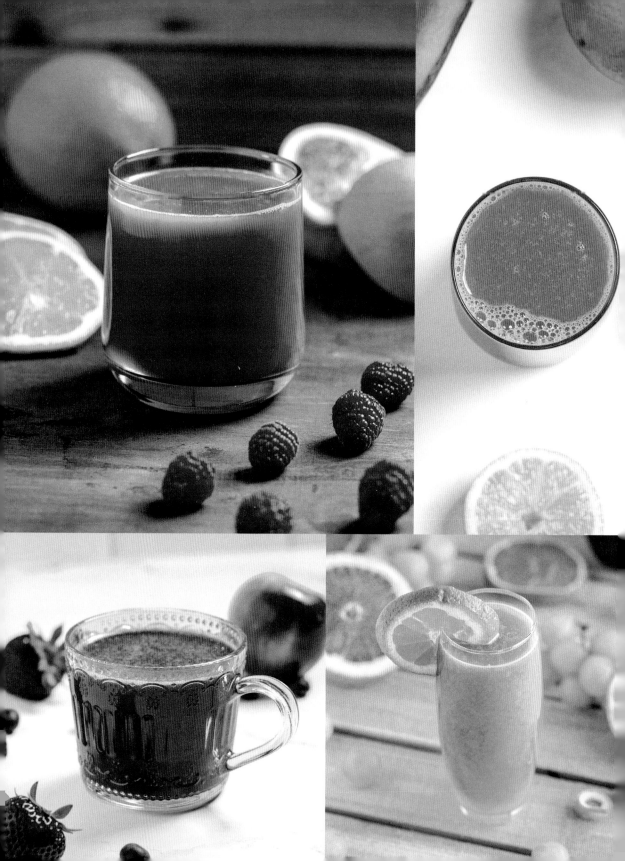

THE SWEET LIFE
FRUIT JUICES

Most juices you find at the grocery store are loaded with added sugars and syrups. Plus, many of the amazing health benefits are lost during heating and processing. When you start making your own juices, it's hard to go back to conventional store-bought juice. Your own juices just taste so much better, and they are filled with so many phytonutrients, vitamins, minerals and health benefits.

This chapter features recipes using fruits you can easily find at the grocery store. I hope you enjoy them as much as I do. You just can't beat the juiciness of fresh fruit!

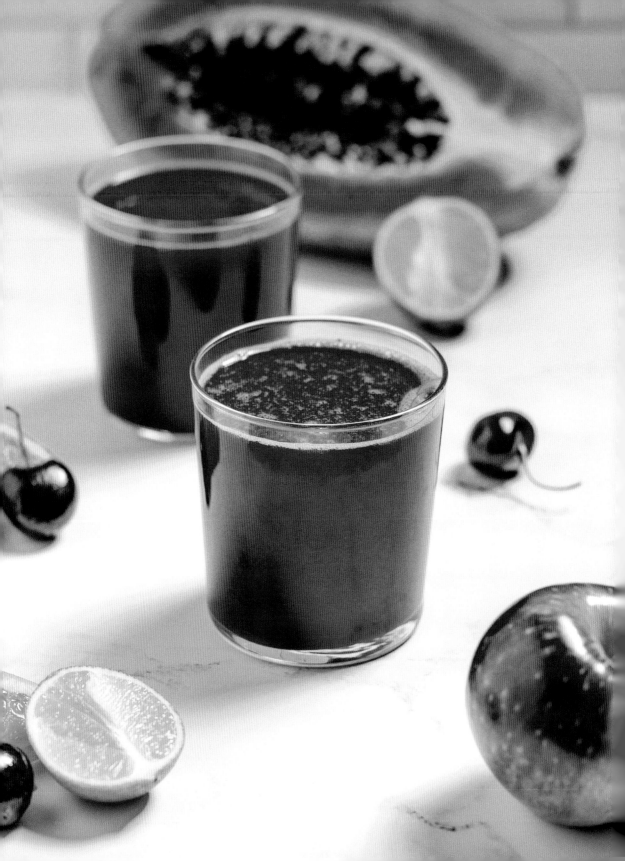

SWEET CHERRY PUNCH

This sweet, slightly citrus-fruity cherry punch is incredibly smooth. I love all the benefits papaya has to offer. I try to incorporate it as much as I can, and when it's added with other fruit, it creates a delectable juice. These fruits are packed with antioxidants and help support your gut health, digestive health and more. Sit back and take a sip . . . your digestive system will thank you.

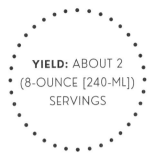

YIELD: ABOUT 2
(8-OUNCE [240-ML])
SERVINGS

GET JUICING!
Wash all your produce and get ready to prep.

Remove the pits and stems from the cherries. Peel the orange. Use a knife to remove the peel from the lime.

There is no need to peel the apple, but you can core it. Nama suggests coring because apple seeds are known to have toxicity; I prefer to core my apples when juicing.

Add the ingredients to the hopper in this order: First layer your softer fruit, then add the apple on top for a smoother juicing process.

Once it's loaded, turn on the juicer and run it until all the ingredients are juiced.

JUICING LINE UP

15 CHERRIES

1 CUP (175 G) DICED
PAPAYA

1 ORANGE

1 LIME

1 APPLE

NOTE: You don't need to cut apples in half, but I prefer to cut mine to make more room in my hopper.

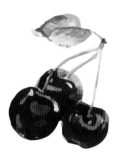

MELLOW COOLER

Stay mellow and cool with this smooth, refreshing juice. This combo can help support healthy skin, fight bloating and more! It's packed with vitamin C and electrolytes, and honeydew is high in water content so it's great for hydration. Whether you're sitting by the pool or want a delicious way to stay hydrated, this is a juice that you will definitely make again and again.

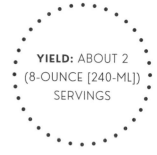

YIELD: ABOUT 2 (8-OUNCE [240-ML]) SERVINGS

JUICING LINE UP

¼ OF A HONEYDEW MELON

1 ENGLISH CUCUMBER

2 LIMES

GET JUICING!

Wash all your produce and get ready to prep.

Remove the seeds and cut the rind off your honeydew. Cut the melon into smaller chunks to fit easily into the hopper. Cut the cucumber into quarters to fit easily in the hopper. Use a knife to remove the peel from the limes, and cut them in half.

Add the ingredients to the hopper in any order you like. Layering doesn't matter for this juice, as the ingredients have a similar firmness to them.

Once it's loaded, turn on the juicer and run it until all the ingredients are juiced.

TIP: Cutting honeydew in half first makes it easier to remove the rind.

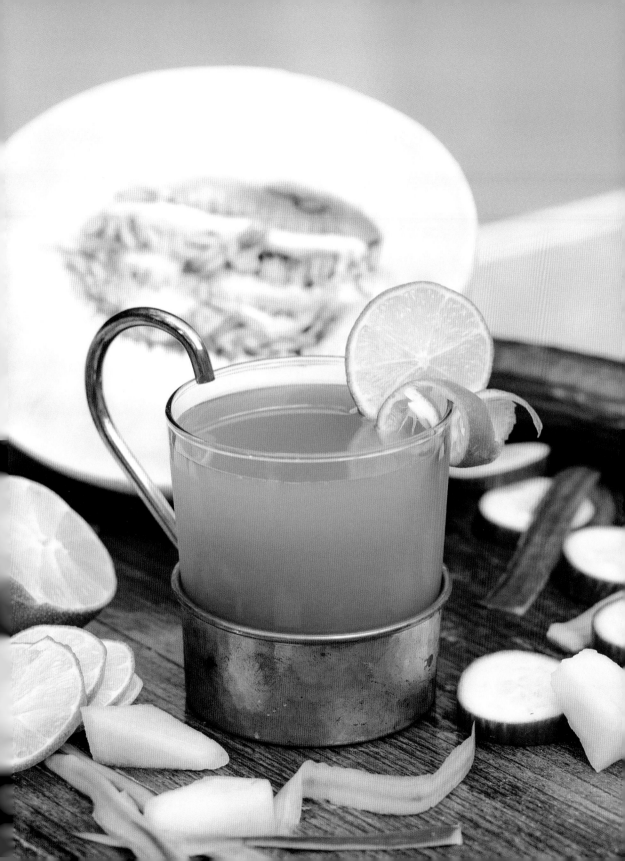

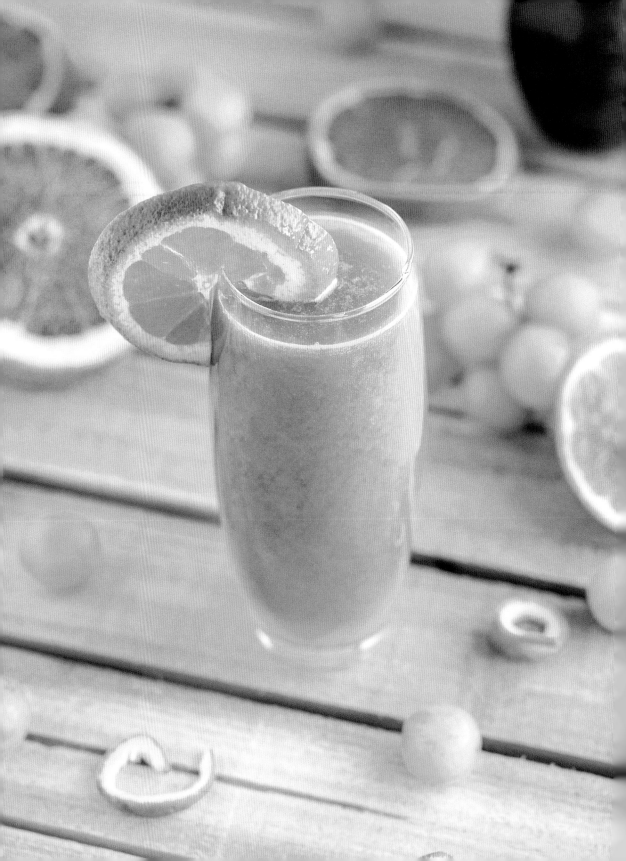

TROPICAL ORCHARD

Support your immune system with this vitamin C–packed juice. This tart citrus punch is a treat and has a subtle sweetness with grapefruit shining through. Please note grapefruit can affect certain medications. Talk to your doctor if you're on medication before consuming grapefruit.

YIELD: ABOUT 2 (8-OUNCE [240-ML]) SERVINGS

GET JUICING!

Wash all your produce and get ready to prep.

Peel the orange and grapefruit. Remove the stems from the grapes. There is no need to peel the apple, but you can core it. Nama suggests coring because apple seeds are known to have toxicity; I prefer to core my apples when juicing.

Add the ingredients to the hopper in this order: First layer your orange and grapefruit, then add the grapes and the apple on top for a smoother juicing process.

Once it's loaded, turn on the juicer and run it until all the ingredients are juiced.

JUICING LINE UP

1 ORANGE

1 GRAPEFRUIT

1 CUP TABLE GRAPES (30 GRAPES)

1 APPLE

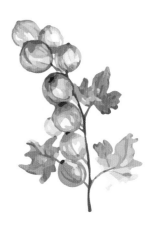

TIP: If you want a less bitter juice, instead of peeling the grapefruit, use a knife to cut off the peel and remove the white pith. I like to keep it on!

CITRUS MELLOW

Mellow out. . . . This juice is another great way to sneak in some papaya. It's smooth with a light tart taste. This juice is packed with so many flavors and, of course, health benefits. These fruits are known to support digestive health, heart health and your metabolism; plus, they have anticancer properties and more! Please note grapefruit can interfere with some medication, always consult with your doctor before consuming.

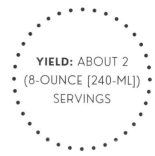

YIELD: ABOUT 2 (8-OUNCE [240-ML]) SERVINGS

• •

GET JUICING!

Wash all your produce and get ready to prep.

Peel the orange, grapefruit and lemon. Use a knife to remove the peel of the mango. Remove the pit from the mango and the apricot.

Add the ingredients to the hopper in this order: First layer your orange, grapefruit and lemon, then add the mango, apricot and papaya on top for a smoother juicing process.

Once it's loaded, turn on the juicer and run it until all the ingredients are juiced.

JUICING LINE UP

1 ORANGE

1 GRAPEFRUIT

½ OF A LEMON

½ OF A MANGO

1 APRICOT

1 CUP (175 G) DICED PAPAYA

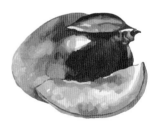

• •

TIP: Cutting the mango in half first and scooping out the "meat" is a great way to quickly get it out without trying to cut it out.

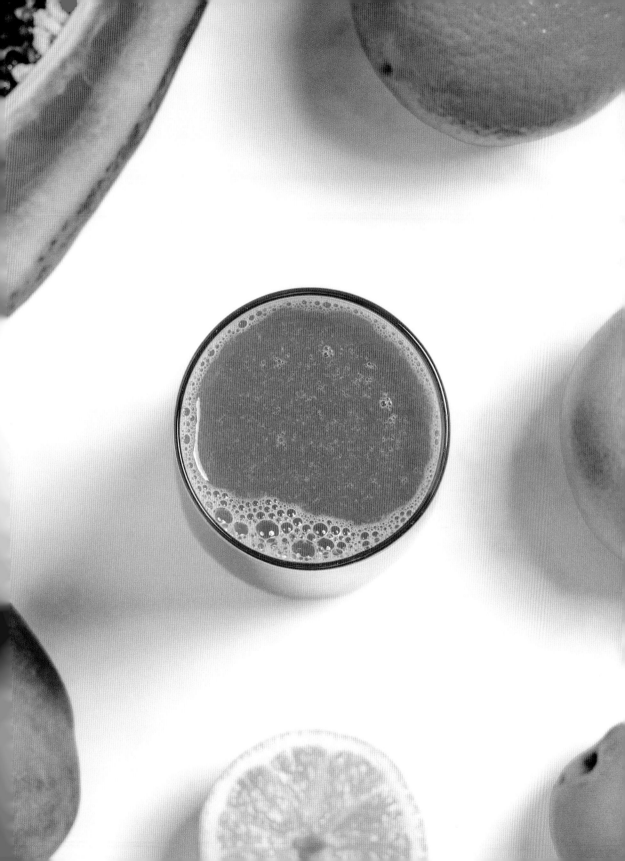

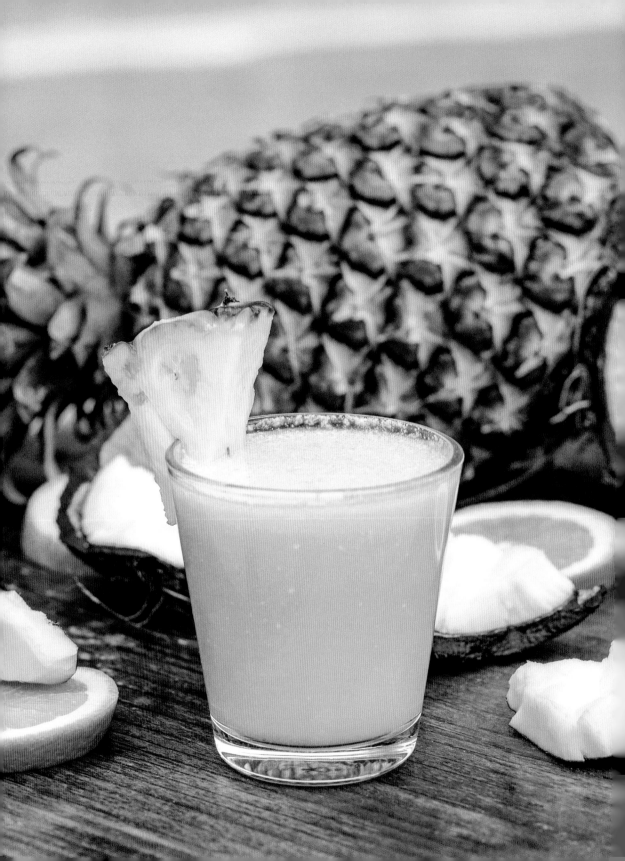

ORANGE–PIÑA COLADA

Hold the alcohol! This is a delicious twist on the classic piña colada. It will have you feeling like you are on vacation. We love to have this dessert-style juice after dinner, sitting on the balcony and pretending we're traveling. These fruits are known to be packed with antioxidants, potassium, vitamin C and more!

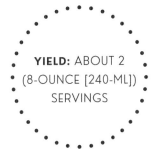

YIELD: ABOUT 2 (8-OUNCE [240-ML]) SERVINGS

GET JUICING!

Wash all your produce and get ready to prep.

Peel the oranges. Remove the crown from the pineapple and remove the skin. I don't core my pineapple; I like to keep it because there are many nutrients found in the core. Once you remove the skin from your pineapple, cut it into small chunks.

Add the ingredients to the hopper in this order: First layer your oranges and pineapple, then add the coconut meat on top for a smoother juicing process.

Once it's loaded, turn on the juicer and run it until all the ingredients are juiced.

JUICING LINE UP

2 ORANGES

½ OF A PINEAPPLE

1 CUP (80 G) COCONUT MEAT

TIPS

- Soak the coconut meat in water for 1 hour beforehand to make it softer to juice.
- The coconut does add some creaminess when juiced; if you see little cream chunks in your juice, it's normal.

HYDRATING PUNCH

Hydrate your brain cells with these brain-supporting, antioxidant and vitamin C–packed fruits! Don't overcomplicate taking care of your health. It can be as simple as replacing a conventional juice from the grocery store with a homemade nutrient-packed juice. No added sugars or syrups here—this is all juicy goodness.

YIELD: ABOUT 2 (8-OUNCE [240-ML]) SERVINGS

GET JUICING!

Wash all your produce and get ready to prep.

Peel the orange. Remove the stem from the pear. Remove the crown from the pineapple and remove the skin. I don't core my pineapple; I like to keep it because there are many nutrients found in the core. Once you remove the skin from your pineapple, cut it into small chunks.

There is no need to peel the apple, but you can core it. Nama suggests coring because apple seeds are known to have toxicity; I prefer to core my apples when juicing.

Add the ingredients to the hopper in this order: First layer your blueberries, then add the orange, pear, pineapple and apple on top for a smoother juicing process.

Once it's loaded, turn on the juicer and run it until all the ingredients are juiced.

JUICING LINE UP

½ CUP (75 G) BLUEBERRIES

1 ORANGE

1 PEAR

¼ OF A PINEAPPLE

½ OF AN APPLE

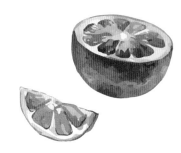

NOTE: Blueberries will add a thicker consistency to the juice.

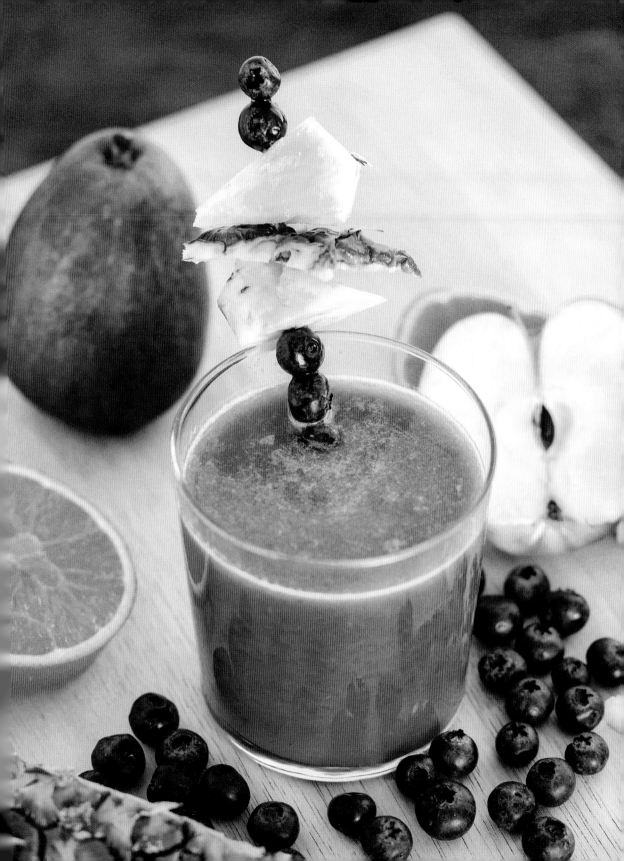

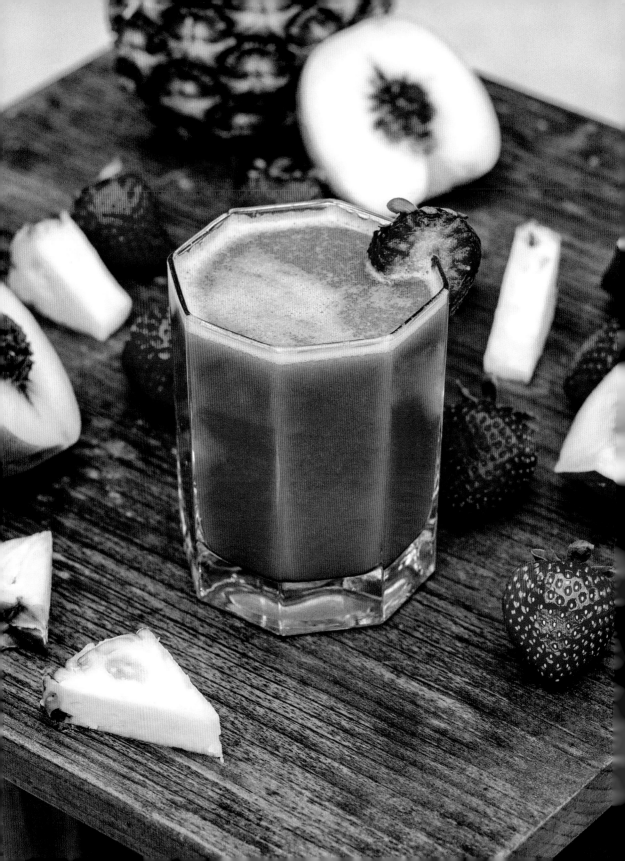

PINEAPPLE BURST

If you're looking for a candy-like juice, this is the one. This juice is such a treat, and what makes it even better is these fruits are known to help support your gut health and so much more! This juice is more on the acidic side with just the right amount of sweetness from the strawberries to give it a balanced fruity flavor.

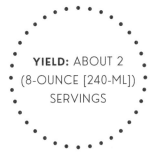

YIELD: ABOUT 2 (8-OUNCE [240-ML]) SERVINGS

GET JUICING!

Wash all your produce and get ready to prep.

Remove the pit from the peach. Cut the peach into smaller pieces. Remove the crown from the pineapple and remove the skin. I don't core my pineapple; I like to keep it because there are many nutrients found in the core. Once you remove the skin from your pineapple, cut it into small chunks.

Add the ingredients to the hopper in this order: First layer your strawberries, then add the peach and pineapple on top for a smoother juicing process.

Once it's loaded, turn on the juicer and run it until all the ingredients are juiced.

JUICING LINE UP

½ LB (226 G) STRAWBERRIES (ABOUT 9)

1 WHITE PEACH

¼ OF A PINEAPPLE

NOTE: You don't have to remove the leaves from the strawberries. They are edible and can be juiced.

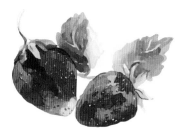

CITRUS CRUSH

Your skin's new crush! Raspberries are known to have antiaging properties and are great for maintaining healthy skin. That makes this juice a great addition to your skin care routine—starting from the inside out! I love switching up my morning juices, and this one is a refreshing citrus blend. Please note grapefruit can interfere with some medication; always consult with your doctor before consuming.

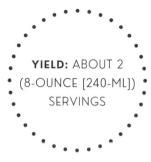

- -

JUICING LINE UP

2 ORANGES

1 GRAPEFRUIT

6 OZ (170 G) RASPBERRIES

GET JUICING!

Wash all your produce and get ready to prep.

Peel the oranges and grapefruit.

Add the ingredients to the hopper in any order you like. Layering doesn't matter for this juice, as the ingredients have a similar softness to them.

Once it's loaded, turn on the juicer and run it until all the ingredients are juiced.

- -

TIP: Don't soak raspberries too long when washing them; they will get mushy.

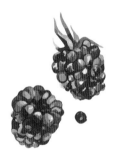

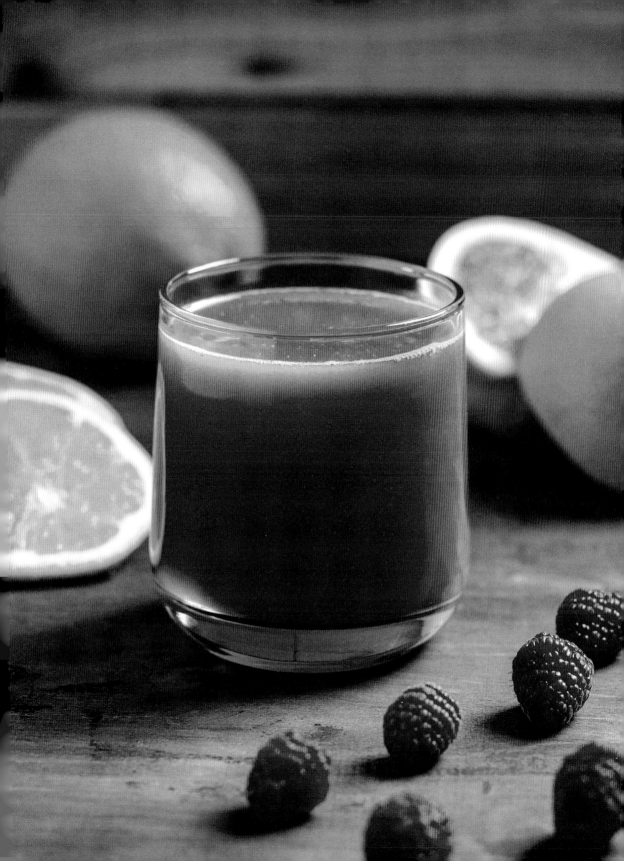

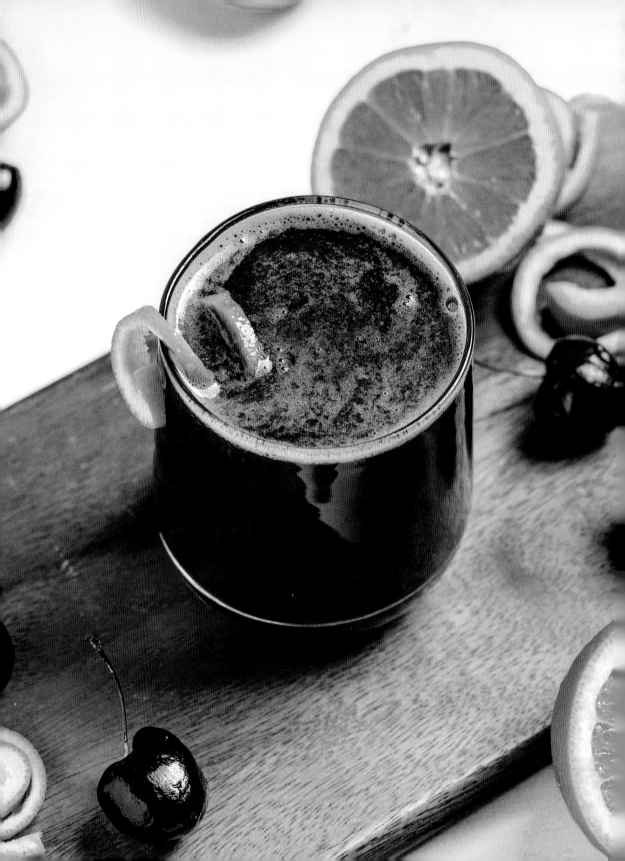

CHERRY-O

A new twist on the classic OJ. Cherries add incredible fruity flavor to this juice and are packed with vitamin C. Cherries also have anti-inflammatory properties and help support your metabolism. This is a great simple juice to add to your rotation.

YIELD: ABOUT 2 (8-OUNCE [240-ML]) SERVINGS

GET JUICING!

Wash all your produce and get ready to prep.

Remove the pits and stems from the cherries. Peel the oranges.

Add the ingredients to the hopper in any order you like. Layering doesn't matter for this juice, as the ingredients have a similar softness to them.

Once it's loaded, turn on the juicer and run it until all the ingredients are juiced.

JUICING LINE UP

24 CHERRIES

4 ORANGES

TIP: I recommend using a cherry pitter to remove pits from cherries. It makes it quicker and easier than cutting out pits with a knife. Do not leave pits in the cherries, as they can damage your juicer.

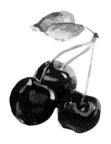

COSMIC HARVEST

I'm feeling berry good with this superfood juice combo. If you haven't tried a Cosmic Crisp apple, you have to give this juice a try. It has the perfect crisp sweet-tart flavor. These fruits are packed with powerful antioxidants and vitamin C, support heart health, are anti-inflammatory and so much more.

YIELD: ABOUT 2 (8-OUNCE [240-ML]) SERVINGS

GET JUICING!

Wash all your produce and get ready to prep.

There is no need to peel the apple, but you can core it. Nama suggests coring because apple seeds are known to have toxicity; I prefer to core my apples when juicing.

Add the ingredients to the hopper in this order: First layer your berries, then add the apple on top for a smoother juicing process.

Once it's loaded, turn on the juicer and run it until all the ingredients are juiced. You will notice that this juice has a thicker consistency because of the berries.

JUICING LINE UP

1 LB (454 G)
STRAWBERRIES

6 OZ (170 G)
BLUEBERRIES

1 COSMIC CRISP APPLE

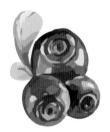

TIP: If you want to save time, keep the leaves on the strawberries. They are edible, have nutrients and can be juiced!

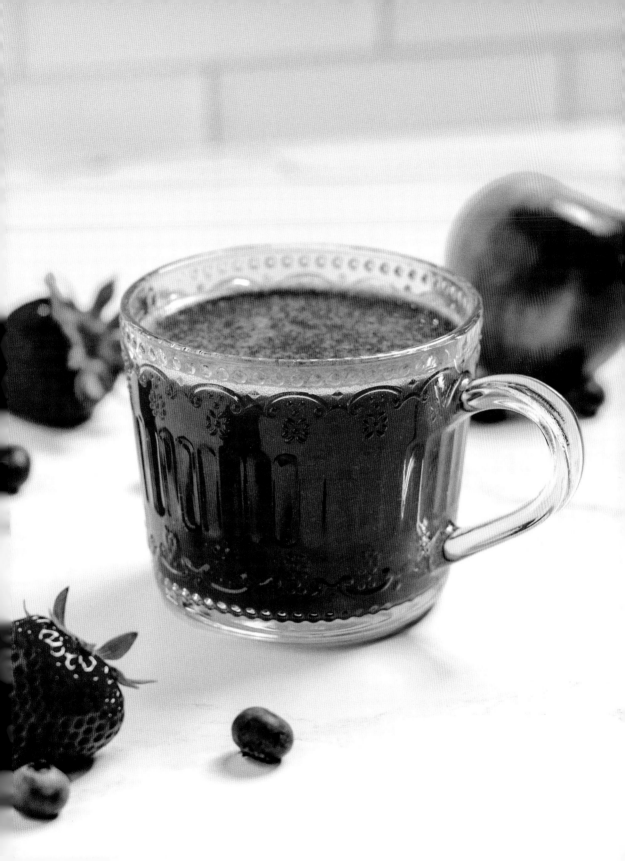

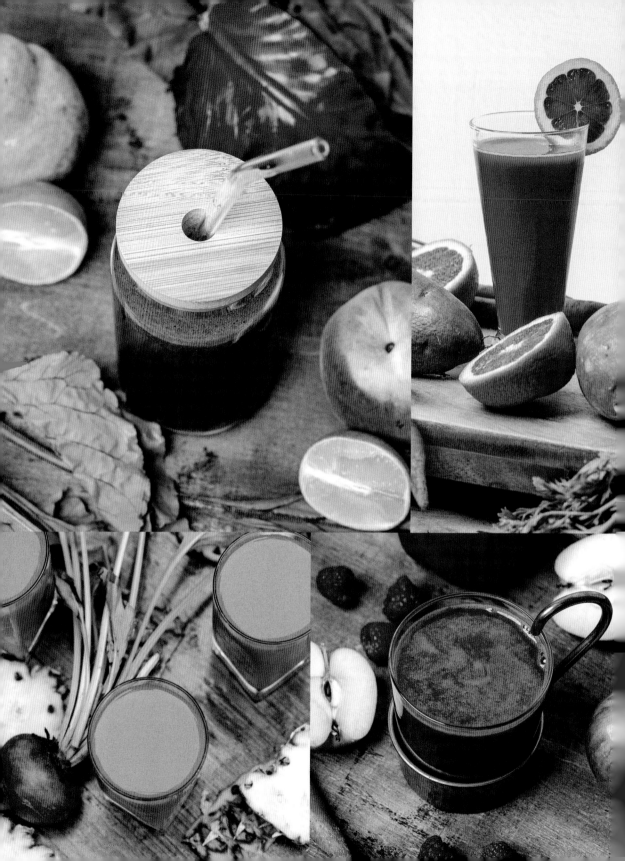

COLORFUL
ENERGIZING JUICES

I love to begin a day with green juice, but we also need to switch up our juice rotation to be sure we are getting all the colors of the rainbow. This chapter includes recipes to help you start your morning with the colors of the rising sun. The juices are filled with a variety of flavors and colors from papayas, oranges, carrots, beets—and even . . . red bell peppers and sweet potatoes! These ingredients support healthy skin and your immune system. They also have anticancer properties and more.

Try these surprising combos. You may find your new favorite juice!

This chapter features recipes using fruits you can easily find at the grocery store. I hope you enjoy them as much as I do. You just can't beat the juiciness of fresh fruit!

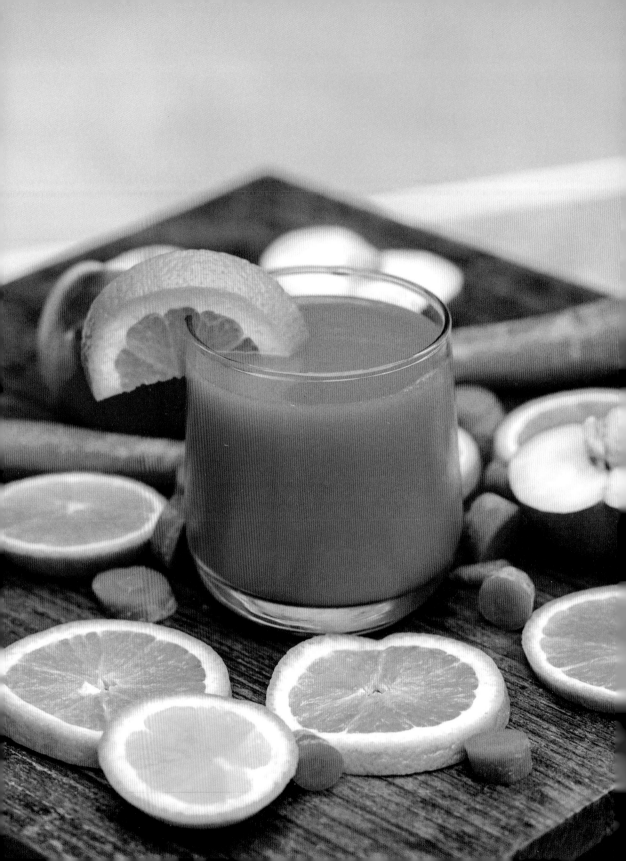

PEACHY C BLAST

I love peaches! Here in Michigan, peach season is short, but we take full advantage when it's here. Peaches are such a great treat to add to your juice. They are rich in antioxidants and add a refreshing, delicate sweet flavor. This is a great summer morning juice that is packed with vitamin C and immune system–supporting properties.

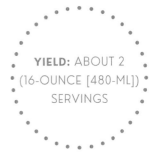

YIELD: ABOUT 2 (16-OUNCE [480-ML]) SERVINGS

GET JUICING!
Wash all your produce and get ready to prep.

Peel the oranges. Remove the pits from the peaches. Remove the tops from the carrots, then cut them into smaller chunks to fit them more easily in your hopper.

Add the ingredients to the hopper in this order: First layer your oranges and peaches, then add the carrots on top for a smoother juicing process.

Once it's loaded, turn on the juicer and run it until all the ingredients are juiced.

JUICING LINE UP

4 CARA CARA OR NAVEL ORANGES

4 WHITE PEACHES

1 LB (454 G) CARROTS

TIP: When selecting peaches, the more fragrant they are, the riper they tend to be.

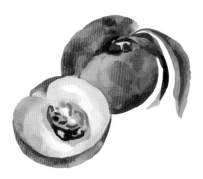

GOLDEN HARVEST

Feeling under the weather? Make sure you nourish and rejuvenate your body by getting in your vitamin C with this tangy, rooty juice. Vitamin C is essential for supporting your immune system, keeping your skin healthy and so much more. Plus, the sweet potato gives this juice a satisfying creaminess.

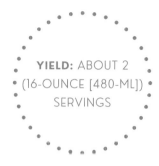

YIELD: ABOUT 2 (16-OUNCE [480-ML]) SERVINGS

GET JUICING!

Wash all your produce and get ready to prep.

Peel the oranges. Remove the tops from the carrots, then cut them into smaller chunks to fit them more easily in your hopper. Cut the sweet potatoes in half to fit easily in the hopper.

Add the ingredients to the hopper in this order: First layer your oranges, then add the carrots and sweet potatoes for a smoother juicing process.

Once it's loaded, turn on the juicer and run it until all the ingredients are juiced.

NOTE: This juice tends to be grainy. You can strain it for a smoother juice.

JUICING LINE UP

4 CARA CARA ORANGES

2 LB (907 G) CARROTS

2 LB (907 G) SWEET POTATOES

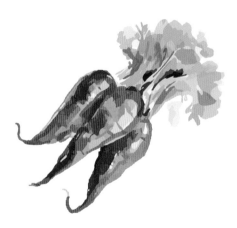

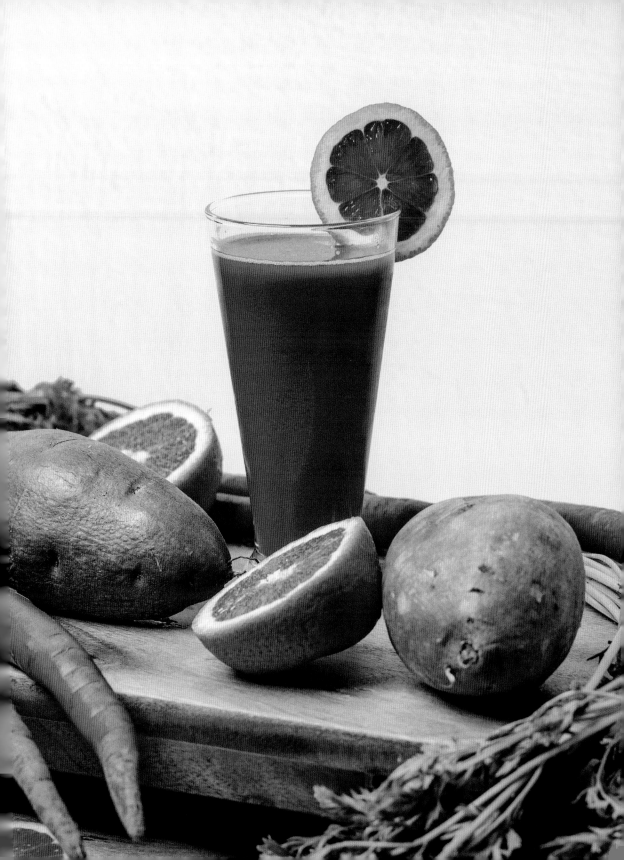

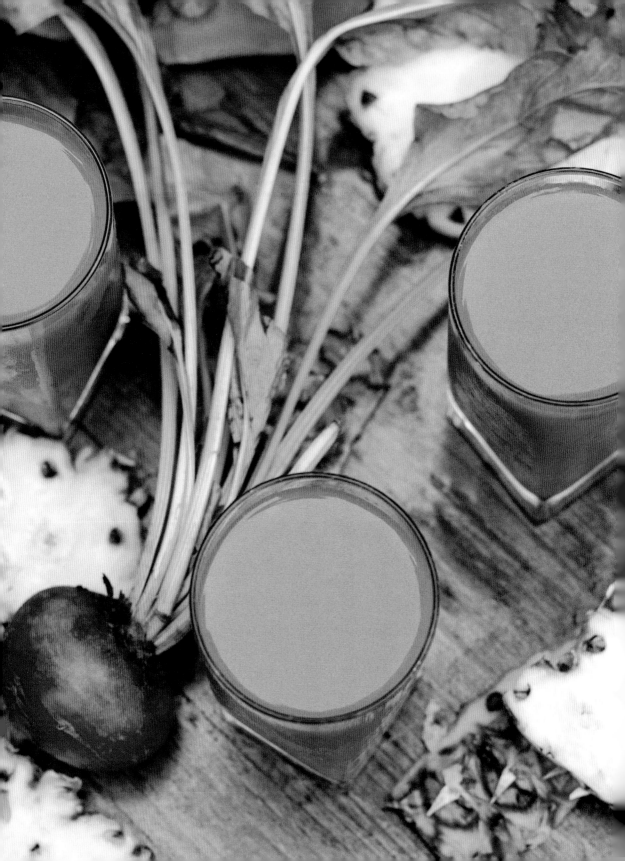

MORNING ZING

This juice provides iron to help support menstruation and the symptoms it comes with; I make it when I need some extra support, especially in the mornings. Pineapple is packed with anti-inflammatory properties and is great for fighting bloating and swelling.

YIELD: ABOUT 2 (16-OUNCE [480-ML]) SERVINGS

GET JUICING!

Wash all your produce and get ready to prep.

Remove the crown from the pineapple and remove the skin. I don't core my pineapple; I like to keep it because there are many nutrients found in the core. Once you remove the skin from your pineapple, cut it into small chunks.

Cut sweet potatoes and beets in half to fit easily in the hopper.

Add the ingredients to the hopper in this order: First layer your pineapple, then add the sweet potatoes and beets on top for a smoother juicing process.

Once it's loaded, turn on the juicer and run it until all the ingredients are juiced.

JUICING LINE UP

1 SMALL PINEAPPLE

2 SWEET POTATOES

2 GOLDEN BEETS

NOTE: Golden beets give this juice a less earthy flavor compared to red beets.

JOHNNY-O SAFARIO

This is a recipe I hold near to my heart. This was one of the last recipes I made for my father-in-law, John, before he passed away after a long battle with cancer. I specifically made this blend for him knowing he loved cherries and was requesting cherry juice during this time. Cherries are known to help support better sleep. I snuck in some purple cabbage and apple, and he loved it! I hope you enjoy it as much as he did.

YIELD: ABOUT 2 (16-OUNCE [480-ML]) SERVINGS

JUICING LINE UP

46 CHERRIES

½ OF A PURPLE CABBAGE

2 COSMIC CRISP APPLES

. . . .

GET JUICING!

Wash all your produce and get ready to prep.

Remove the stems and pits from the cherries. Remove a few of the outer leaves from the cabbage, including any that are damaged or wilted. Cut it into pieces to fit easily in the hopper.

There is no need to peel the apples, but you can core them. Nama suggests coring because apple seeds are known to have toxicity; I prefer to core my apples when juicing.

Add the ingredients to the hopper in this order: First layer your cherries, then add the cabbage and apples on top for a smoother juicing process.

Once it's loaded, turn on the juicer and run it until all the ingredients are juiced.

. . . .

TIP: I recommend using a cherry pitter to remove pits from cherries. It makes it quicker and easier. Do not leave pits in the cherries, as they can damage your juicer.

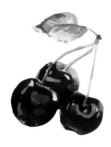

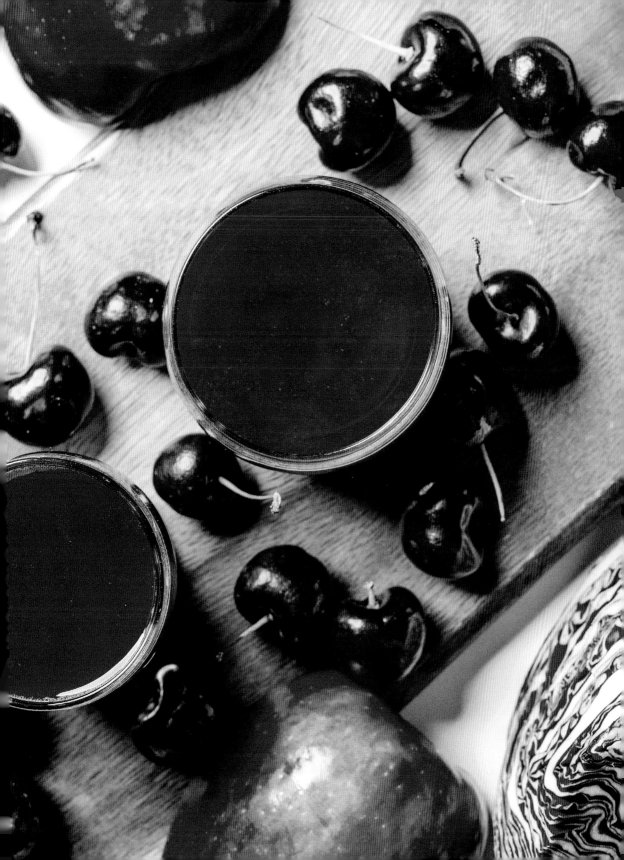

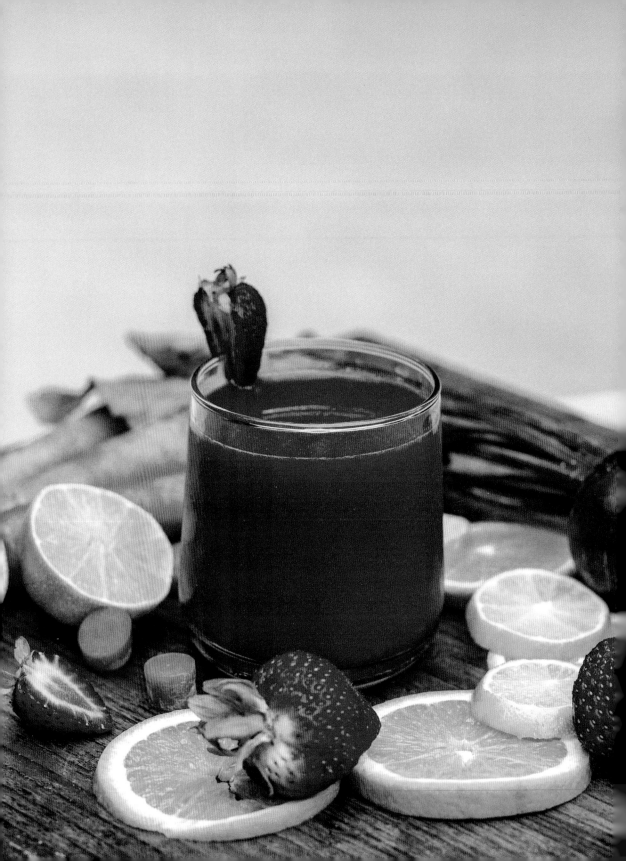

FESTIVE SOL

There's nothing better than a cold drink on a hot, sunny day. Well, I can think of one thing: making sure it's packed with fruit and veggies that have much-desired health benefits. This juice supports healthy blood flow, heart health, skin health and more. It is sunshine in a cup!

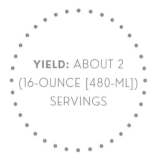

YIELD: ABOUT 2 (16-OUNCE [480-ML]) SERVINGS

GET JUICING!

Wash all your produce and get ready to prep.

Peel the oranges. Use a knife to remove the peels from the limes. Remove the tops from the carrots, then cut them into smaller chunks to fit them more easily in your hopper. Remove the beet tops from your beet.

Add the ingredients to the hopper in this order: First layer your strawberries, then add the oranges and limes (if using). Add the carrots and beet on top for a smoother juicing process.

Once it's loaded, turn on the juicer and run it until all the ingredients are juiced.

JUICING LINE UP

32 STRAWBERRIES

2 ORANGES

2 LIMES, OPTIONAL

14 CARROTS

1 MEDIUM RED BEET

TIP: You can keep the tops of strawberries on; the leaves are edible.

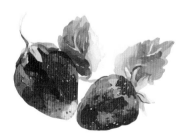

PEPPERY DELIGHT

People are always surprised when I tell them bell peppers and tomatoes are great add-ins for juices. Simple and delicious! I know you may be skeptical, but by now you know I wouldn't say something is good unless I truly think it's good. This juice is a delight with a punch of vitamin C and immune system–supporting fruits and veggies.

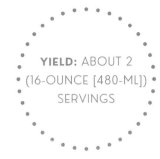

YIELD: ABOUT 2 (16-OUNCE [480-ML]) SERVINGS

· ·

GET JUICING!

Wash all your produce and get ready to prep.

Peel the oranges. Remove the seeds from the bell peppers.

There is no need to peel the apple, but you can core it. Nama suggests coring because apple seeds are known to have toxicity; I prefer to core my apples when juicing.

Add the ingredients to the hopper in this order: First layer your oranges, then add the cherries, tomatoes, bell peppers and apple on top for a smoother juicing process.

Once it's loaded, turn on the juicer and run it until all the ingredients are juiced.

JUICING LINE UP

4 ORANGES

20 CHERRIES

2 ROMA TOMATOES

2 RED, ORANGE OR YELLOW BELL PEPPERS

1 COSMIC CRISP APPLE

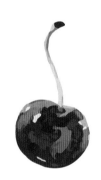

· ·

NOTE: I prefer to take out the seeds, but you can leave the seeds in the bell peppers; it will give the juice a more peppery taste to it.

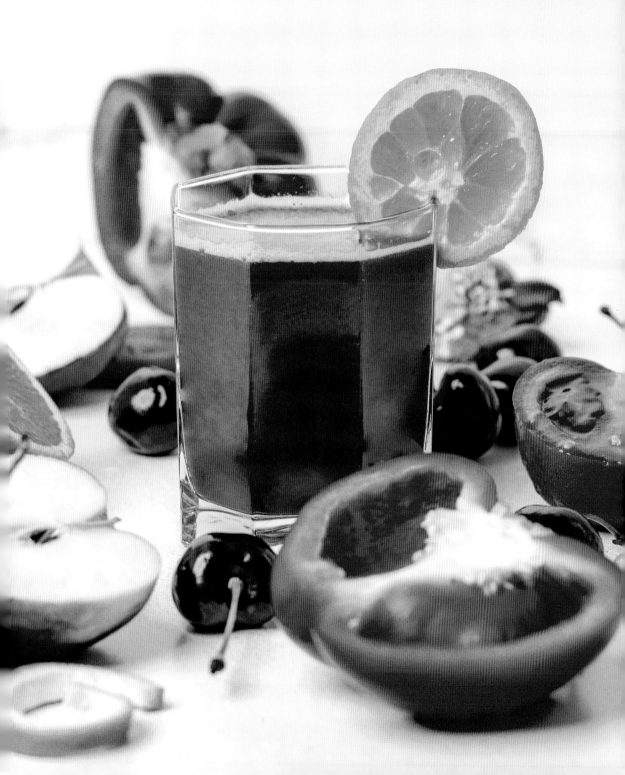

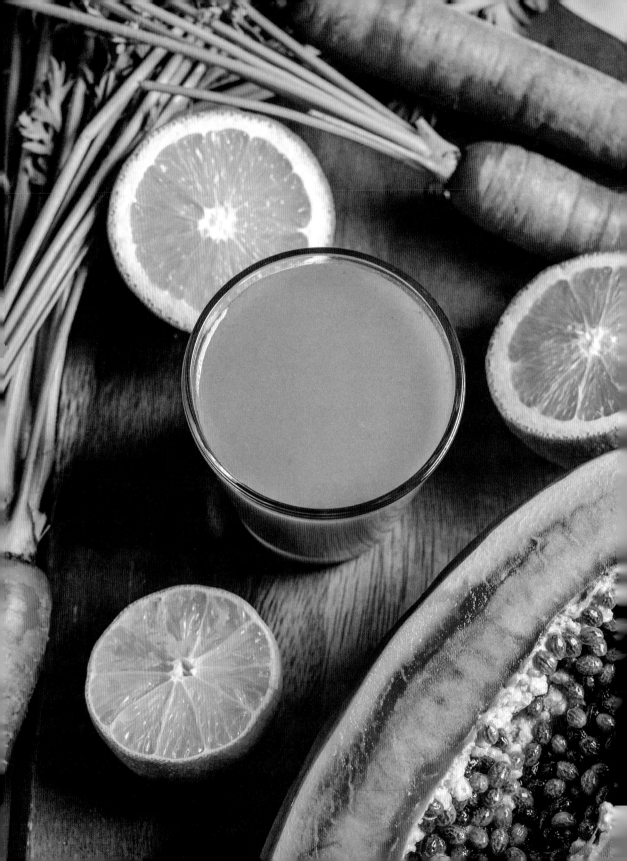

WAKE-UP CALL

I cannot say this enough: papaya does wonders to all things digestive. If you are struggling with your digestive health, constipation or bloating, incorporate it into your juice rotations. It is packed with powerful digestive enzymes. I don't love papaya on its own, but it's amazing in this juice. And the benefits I've seen from drinking it have been so incredible for my digestive system. I see why people praise the benefits so much. I hope you enjoy this combo!

GET JUICING!

Wash all your produce and get ready to prep.

Peel the oranges. Use a knife to remove the peel from the limes. Remove the tops from the carrots, then cut them into smaller chunks to fit them more easily in your hopper.

Add the ingredients to the hopper in this order: First layer your oranges and limes, then add the papaya and carrots on top for a smoother juicing process.

Once it's loaded, turn on the juicer and run it until all the ingredients are juiced.

NOTE: A half of a small papaya is about 5 cups (700 g) of cubed papaya.

YIELD: ABOUT 2 (16-OUNCE [480-ML]) SERVINGS

JUICING LINE UP

4 ORANGES

2 LIMES

5 CUPS (700 G) CUBED PAPAYA

2 LB (907 G) CARROTS

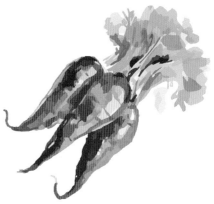

SWEET SUMMER

Summertime means lots of sun. . . . Make sure you are protecting your skin from the inside out! These fruits and veggies are known to have antiaging properties and are packed with vitamins and minerals that are essential for our well-being. Don't let all the veggies in this juice fool you into thinking it isn't sweet. Because it's sweet! Red bell peppers are the sweetest out of all the colors, and they have more vitamin C than oranges and carrots!

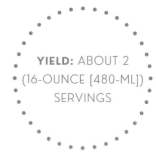

YIELD: ABOUT 2 (16-OUNCE [480-ML]) SERVINGS

. . . .

GET JUICING!

Wash all your produce and get ready to prep.

Remove the seeds from the bell pepper. There is no need to peel the apples, but you can core them. Nama suggests coring because apple seeds are known to have toxicity; I prefer to core my apples when juicing.

Remove the beet tops from your beet. Remove the tops from the carrots, then cut them into smaller chunks to fit them more easily in your hopper.

Add the ingredients to the hopper in this order: First layer your raspberries, then add the bell pepper, apples, beet and carrots on top for a smoother juicing process.

Once it's loaded, turn on the juicer and run it until all the ingredients are juiced.

JUICING LINE UP

1 PINT (312 G) RASPBERRIES

1 RED BELL PEPPER

2 APPLES

1 MEDIUM RED BEET

10 CARROTS

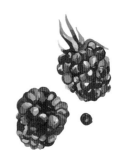

. . . .

TIP: Removing the seeds from the bell pepper gives the juice a less peppery taste to it.

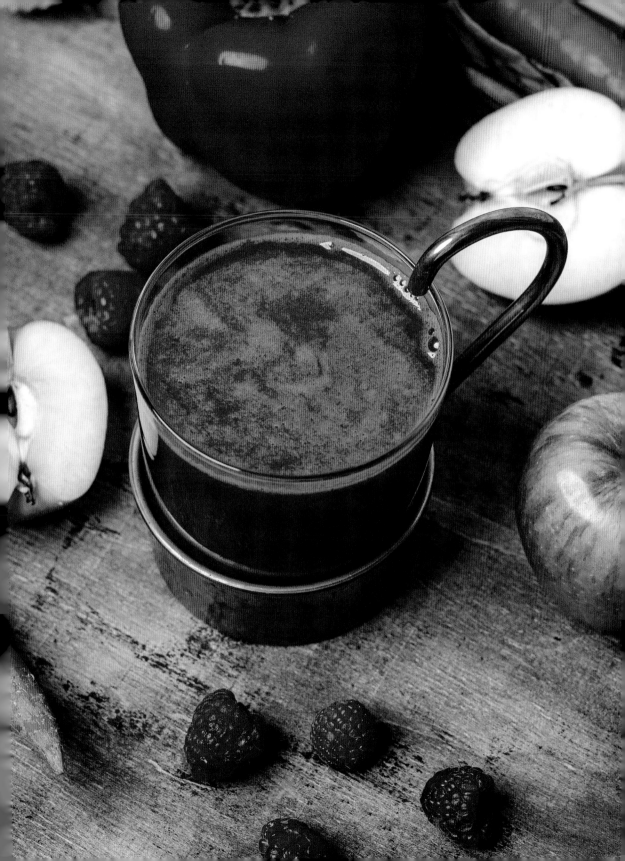

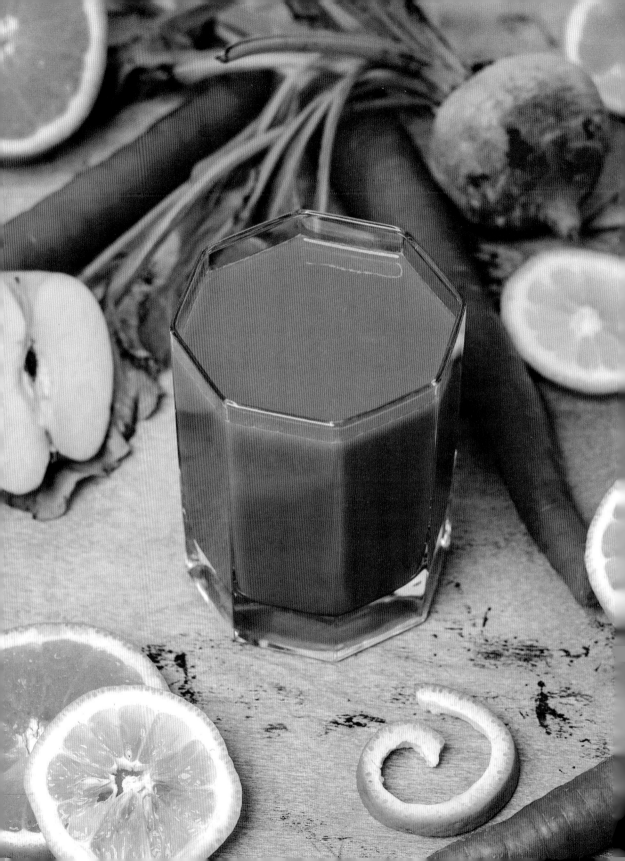

BEET BOOST

Low on iron? Want to support your eye health? Boost your body during a workout? Support healthy liver function? I can go on and on. Try this twist on the classic ABC juice. I'm not the biggest fan of red beets, so I like to use golden beets in my recipes to switch it up. They have a less earthy flavor that doesn't overpower the juice but still adds the amazing benefits. This juice is tangy-sweet and is great for kids, too!

YIELD: ABOUT 2 (16-OUNCE [480-ML]) SERVINGS

· ·

GET JUICING!

Wash all your produce and get ready to prep.

Peel the oranges and lemons. Remove the tops from the carrots, then cut them into smaller chunks to fit them more easily in your hopper.

There is no need to peel the apple, but you can core it. Nama suggests coring because apple seeds are known to have toxicity; I prefer to core my apples when juicing.

Remove the beet tops from your beets.

Add the ingredients to the hopper in this order: First layer your oranges and lemons, then add the carrots, apple and beets on top for a smoother juicing process.

Once it's loaded, turn on the juicer and run it until all the ingredients are juiced.

JUICING LINE UP

4 ORANGES

2 LEMONS

2 LB (907 G) CARROTS

1 APPLE

2 GOLDEN BEETS

· ·

NOTE: You can use red beets in place of golden beets; it will just have a more earthy flavor.

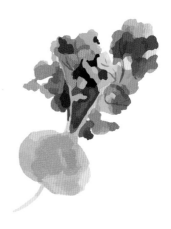

PURPLE JEWEL

Support your gut health and help balance your hormones with this fruit and veggie combo. Purple cabbage can be tough to get into your lifestyle, and it has a strong taste that not everyone likes. This juice is super smooth and is a great way to incorporate it!

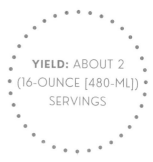

YIELD: ABOUT 2 (16-OUNCE [480-ML]) SERVINGS

. . . .

GET JUICING!

Wash all your produce and get ready to prep.

Remove the pits from the peaches. Use a knife to remove the peels from the limes. Remove the stems from the pears. Remove a few of the outer leaves from the cabbage, including any that are damaged or wilted. Cut it into pieces to fit easily in the hopper. Remove the beet tops from your beet.

Add the ingredients to the hopper in this order: First layer your peaches, then add the limes, pears and purple cabbage. Add the beet on top for a smoother juicing process.

Once it's loaded, turn on the juicer and run it until all the ingredients are juiced.

JUICING LINE UP

4 WHITE PEACHES

2 LIMES

2 PEARS

½ OF A PURPLE CABBAGE

1 SMALL RED BEET

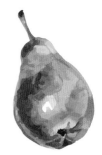

. . . .

TIP: For easier washing, cut cabbages in half. I spray them with a veggie wash (page 13), then rinse them.

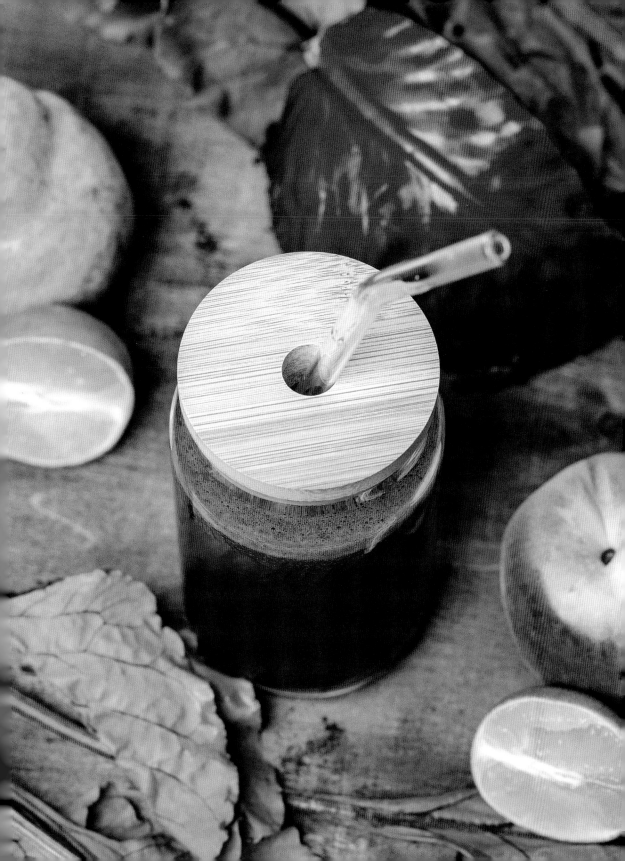

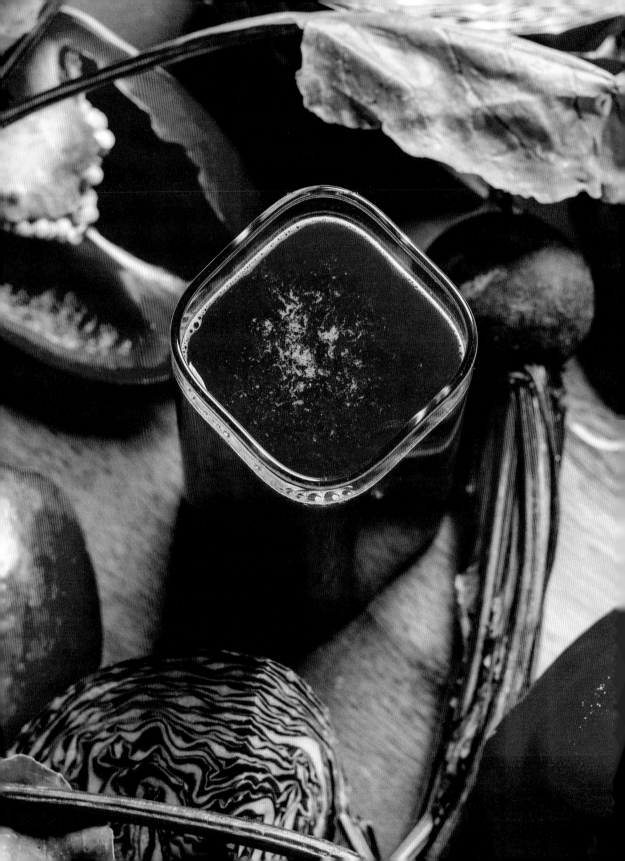

FOREVER YOUNG

What's your skin care routine? That's a question I get constantly. I use simple, natural face oils with rose hips and Moroccan argan oil, but I also make sure I'm nourishing my body from the inside out with juice every morning. I truly believe that great skin starts from what you consume every day. Slow down your skin's aging with these fruits and veggies that support healthy skin and have known antiaging properties.

· ·

GET JUICING!

Wash all your produce and get ready to prep.

Cut the bell pepper in half, and remove the seeds. There is no need to peel the apples, but you can core them. Nama suggests coring because apple seeds are known to have toxicity; I prefer to core my apples when juicing.

Remove a few of the outer leaves from the cabbage, including any that are damaged or wilted. Cut it into pieces to fit easily in the hopper. Remove the beet tops from your beet. Cut the beet in half.

Add the ingredients to the hopper in this order: First layer your bell pepper, then add the apples, cabbage and beet on top for a smoother juicing process.

Once it's loaded, turn on the juicer and run it until all the ingredients are juiced.

· ·

TIP: For easier washing, cut the cabbage in half. I spray it with veggie wash (page 13), then rinse it.

YIELD: ABOUT 2 (16-OUNCE [480-ML]) SERVINGS

JUICING LINE UP

1 RED BELL PEPPER

3 APPLES

1 PURPLE CABBAGE

1 SMALL RED BEET

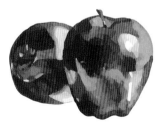

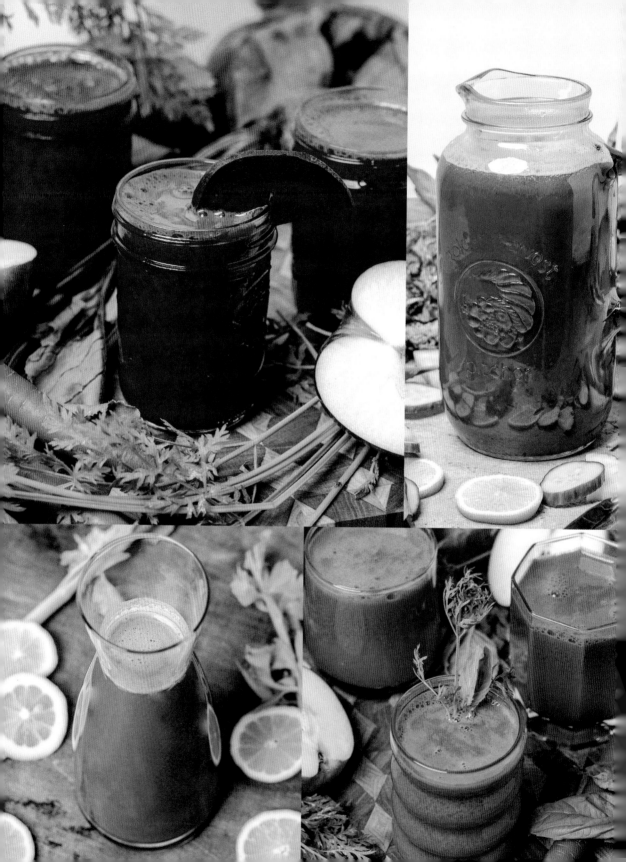

JUICY JUICES FOR DAYS
BATCH JUICING

I love drinking juice fresh, and drinking your juice right after you make it is ideal. It maximizes the number of nutrients you consume. But there are some weeks when I just don't have time to make fresh juice every day.

If you've been following along on social media, you know I love sharing a good batch juice recipe. Batch juicing is so easy and enjoyable in my Nama J2. I created these recipes to help everyone who needs to prep for the week and save time. I hope they help make it easy for you to maintain juicing as a consistent part of your day-to-day life.

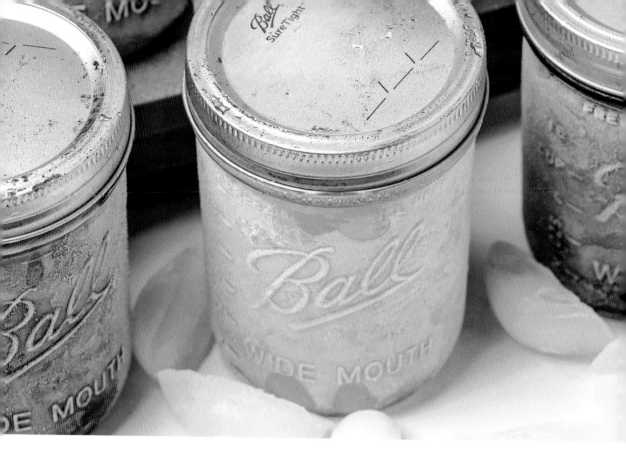

Tips for Freezing Juices

- Cold-pressed juices last for up to 72 hours nutrient-wise. Make sure you drink yours within the 72 hours or freeze them.

- Choose durable containers that are for freezing. I use glass mason jars. They're great for freezing, and I have never had one break on me from being in the freezer.

- Liquid expands when it freezes. Leave a 1-inch (2.5-cm) space at the top of your jar. For wide-mouth mason jars, make sure to fill at or below the lid line. For regular mason jars, fill below the curved "neck" of the jar. Then just top your jars with lids and you are ready to freeze them!

- Take your juice out of the freezer 18 to 20 hours before you plan on drinking it, then let it thaw out in the fridge.

- Do not run your juice container under hot water to thaw it out. The sudden temperature can cause your jar to burst.

- I don't store my juices in the freezer for more than a month. They always get consumed before then!

Tips for Batch Juicing with a J2

- Remember, cold-pressed juices last for up to 72 hours. If you won't be drinking them within that time, freeze them.

- Whether you are storing your juice in the fridge or freezing it, be sure to use sturdy containers. I prefer glass jars with airtight lids.

- Most of my recipes feature fruits and veggies that are easy to find. To keep batching economical, pay attention to sales at your local grocery store. Buy ingredients when they are in season, and buy in bulk when prices are lower.

- Make room in your fridge and freezer before you juice, so you aren't struggling to make room once you are done juicing.

- Have multiple cutting boards and bowls at the ready. Make sure you have ample room to cut fruit and veggies. Have a bowl for finished produce and a second bowl for the skin, peels and cores that you won't be juicing.

- Cut up your celery, ginger, kale, pineapple and any other fibrous or stringy produce for a smoother juicing process.

- Cut produce fits in your hopper more easily, allowing you to have more of that hands-free experience.

If you plan on drinking your juice within 72 hours . . .

You can store it in the fridge.

Fill the container all the way to the top to reduce oxidizing.

Label your juice with the date you made it so you can easily keep track of how long it has been in the fridge.

If you plan on drinking your juice after 72 hours . . .

You can cut your recipe in half and, if you have the ingredients on hand, juice the second half later in the week.

Freeze your juice, and be sure to leave space in your container.

Label your juice with the date you made it so you can easily keep track of how long it has been in the freezer.

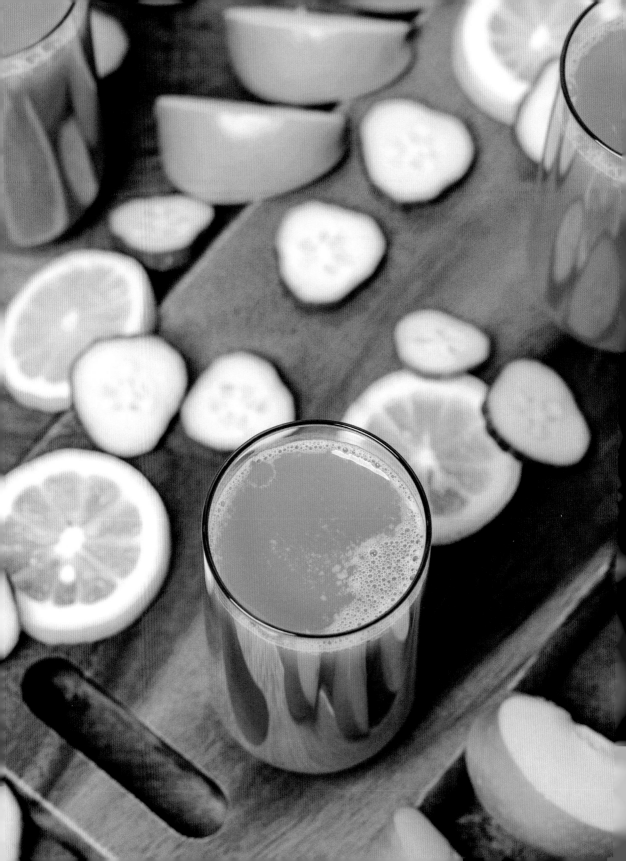

GLOWING GREEN JUICE

Looking for an easy, delicious, healthy way to stay hydrated? This is it! Cucumbers are known to have many health benefits, such as promoting healthy skin, being packed with antioxidants and helping with bloating! The apples and lemon give this blend a refreshing sweet taste. You'll be reaching for this on hot summer days. Batch juicing is so easy with the Nama J2 juicer. Load and go, and you'll have multiple servings in minutes.

• •

GET JUICING!

Wash all your produce and get ready to prep.

Peel the lemons and cut them in half. Cut the cucumbers into quarters to fit easily in the hopper.

I like to peel my ginger with a potato peeler, but you can leave it unpeeled if you prefer. Cut the ginger into smaller pieces for a smoother juicing process.

There is no need to peel the apples, but you can core them. Nama suggests coring because apple seeds are known to have toxicity; I prefer to core my apples when juicing.

Add the ingredients to the hopper in this order: First layer your lemons, then add the cucumbers, ginger (if using) and apples.

Once it's loaded, turn on the juicer and run it until all the ingredients are juiced.

Pour your juice into 16-ounce (480-ml) containers for seven servings. Fill them all the way to the top if storing in the fridge, and leave space in the container if you plan on freezing.

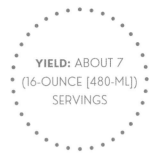

YIELD: ABOUT 7 (16-OUNCE [480-ML]) SERVINGS

JUICING LINE UP

3 LEMONS

12 ENGLISH CUCUMBERS

1 (2-INCH [5-CM]) PIECE OF GINGER, OPTIONAL

3 LARGE GREEN APPLES

• • • • • • • • • • • •

TIP: Make sure to follow Nama's suggested layering to optimize the juicing experience. Softer fruits and veggies on the bottom, and harder fruits and veggies on top. This will make batch juicing smoother.

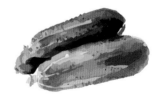

GREEN FUEL

This juice went viral when I posted it on social media. So many people loved it and for good reason. It's packed with so many nutrient-dense fruits and veggies that are known to have anti-inflammatory properties, support your gut health, promote healthy skin and hair, be rich in anti-oxidants and support your metabolism. I had so many people reach out and tell me this combo was so easy and delicious that even their kids were enjoying it. When kids enjoy something with this many greens, you know it's a keeper.

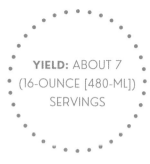

YIELD: ABOUT 7 (16-OUNCE [480-ML]) SERVINGS

GET JUICING!

Wash your leafy greens and other produce, and get ready to prep.

Peel the lemons and cut them in half. Cut the cucumbers into quarters to fit easily in the hopper. Remove the crown from the pineapples and remove the skin. I don't core my pineapple; I like to keep it because there are many nutrients found in the core. Once you remove the skin from your pineapple, cut it into small chunks.

Add the ingredients to the hopper in this order: First layer your leafy greens and lemons, then add the cucumbers and pineapples on top for a smoother juicing process. Once it's loaded, turn on the juicer and run it until all the ingredients are juiced.

Pour your juice into 16-ounce (480-ml) containers for seven servings. Fill them all the way to the top if storing in the fridge, and leave space in the container if you plan on freezing.

JUICING LINE UP

4 PACKED CUPS (320 G) KALE

8 PACKED CUPS (280 G) SPINACH

4 LEMONS

8 ENGLISH CUCUMBERS

2 PINEAPPLES

TIPS

- I like to use spinach that has stems on it; I personally think it juices better.
- Kale can be stringier; if you prefer, you can chop the leaves for a smoother juicing experience.

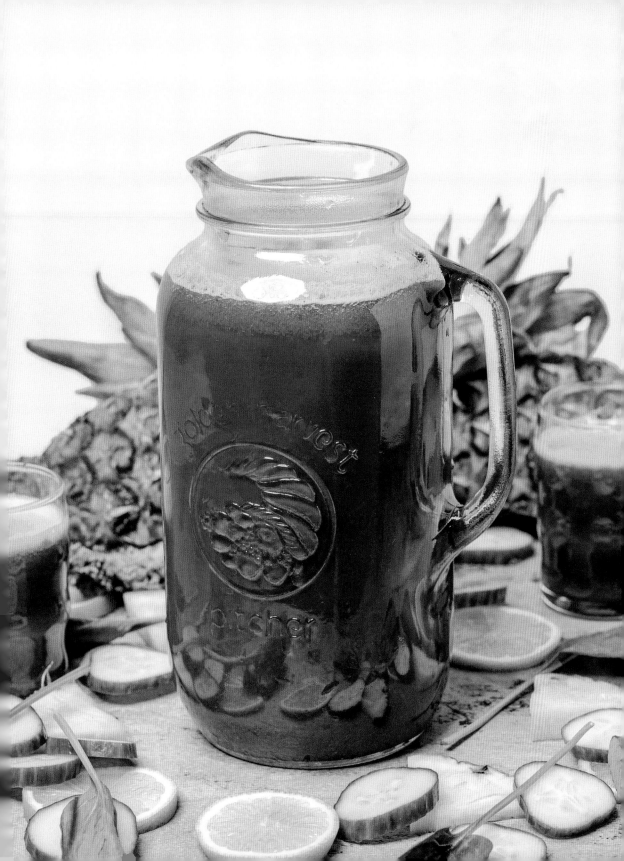

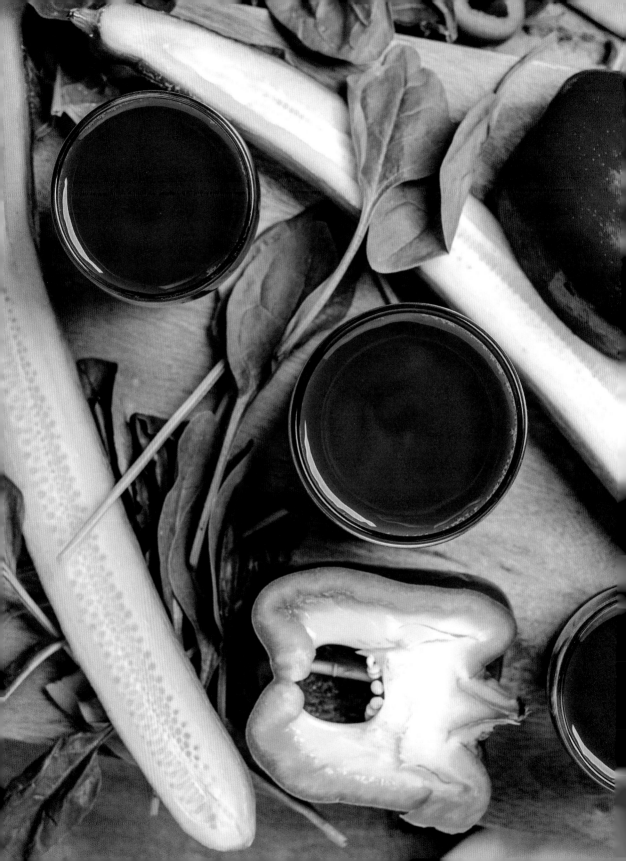

GARDEN PARTY

There's no party like a garden party! I created this recipe inspired by my in-laws' beautiful garden and the simple ingredients you can grow. Throw in some apples, and it's a party. Bell peppers are often forgotten as produce that can be juiced. They are packed with vitamin C and antioxidants; they also support the immune system and more. This is a great way I make sure I get bell peppers in, along with the rest of these nutrient-dense fruits and veggies. This juice is on the veggie-tasting side, flavorful and refreshing with a subtle sweetness to it.

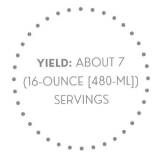

YIELD: ABOUT 7 (16-OUNCE [480-ML]) SERVINGS

JUICING LINE UP

14 PACKED CUPS (490 G) SPINACH

7 ENGLISH CUCUMBERS

4 BELL PEPPERS

6 APPLES

GET JUICING!

Wash your leafy greens and other produce, and get ready to prep.

Remove any wilted spinach leaves. Cut the cucumbers into quarters to fit easily in the hopper. Remove the seeds from the bell peppers.

There is no need to peel the apples, but you can core them. Nama suggests coring because apple seeds are known to have toxicity; I prefer to core my apples when juicing.

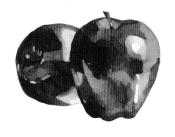

Add the ingredients to the hopper in this order: First layer your spinach, then add the cucumbers, bell peppers and apples on top for a smoother juicing process.

Once it's loaded, turn on the juicer and run it until all the ingredients are juiced.

Pour your juice into 16-ounce (480-ml) containers for seven servings. Fill them all the way to the top if storing in the fridge, and leave space in the container if you plan on freezing.

TIP: I prefer to remove them, but you don't need to remove the seeds from the bell peppers before juicing. It will give the juice a more peppery flavor if you keep them in.

EARLY HARVEST

Don't forget about sweet potatoes! Sweet potatoes are great for juicing and have many health benefits such as supporting the health of your gut, vision and immune system. This rooty blend also supports healthy blood flow. Enjoy the simple, sweet goodness of this juice.

YIELD: ABOUT 7 (16-OUNCE [480-ML]) SERVINGS

GET JUICING!
Wash all your produce and get ready to prep.

Peel the lemons and cut them in half. Remove the tops from the carrots, then cut them into smaller chunks to fit them more easily in your hopper. Cut the sweet potatoes into quarters to fit into the hopper. Remove the tops from your beets.

Add the ingredients to the hopper in this order: First layer your lemons, then add the carrots, sweet potatoes and beets on top for a smoother juicing process.

Once it's loaded, turn on the juicer and run it until all the ingredients are juiced.

Pour your juice into 16-ounce (480-ml) containers for seven servings. Fill them all the way to the top if storing in the fridge, and leave space in the container if you plan on freezing.

JUICING LINE UP

3 LEMONS

6 LB (2.7 KG) CARROTS

9 LB (4 KG) SWEET POTATOES

2 SMALL GOLDEN BEETS

TIP: For a smoother juice, strain this combo. The carrots and sweet potatoes can be grainy.

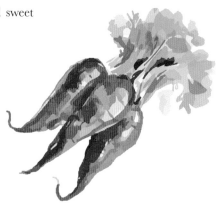

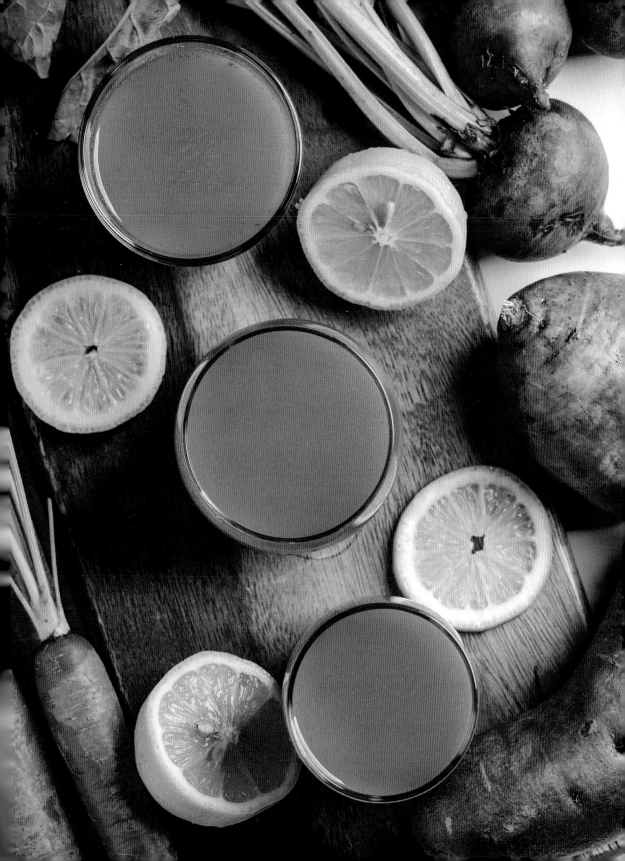

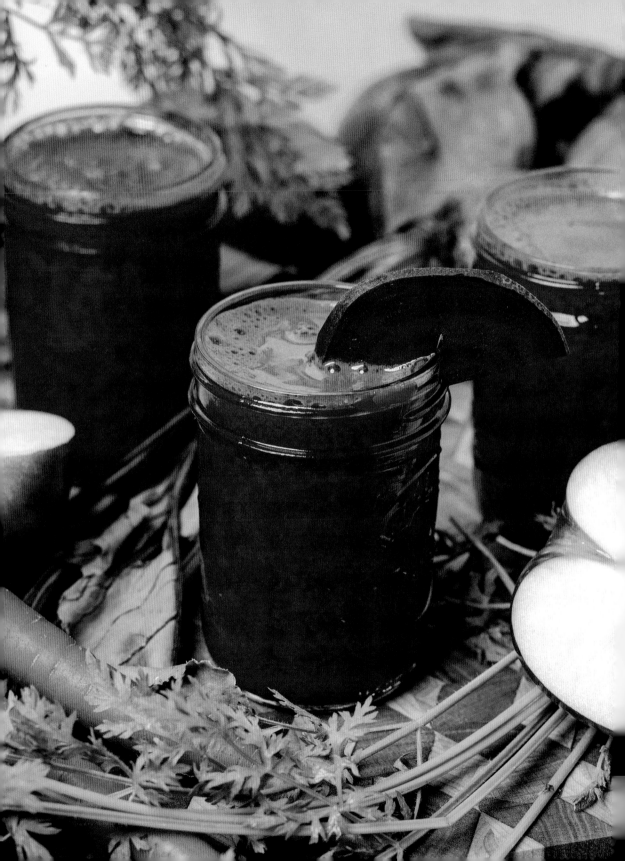

SIMPLY ABC

ABC juice was my mom's signature juice while growing up. . . . I wouldn't really call it ABC juice though. It was mostly beet juice with a splash of apple and carrot. I'm exaggerating, but that's how it felt in my kid-mind. I made my own version of this childhood staple. The fruits and veggies are full of benefits, such as supporting healthy liver function and menstruation. This juice is packed with iron and supports healthy blood flow, healthy vision and more!

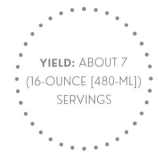

YIELD: ABOUT 7 (16-OUNCE [480-ML]) SERVINGS

JUICING LINE UP

5 COSMIC CRISP APPLES

4 BEETS

10 LB (4.5 KG) CARROTS

GET JUICING!

Wash all your produce and get ready to prep.

There is no need to peel the apples, but you can core them. Nama suggests coring because apple seeds are known to have toxicity; I prefer to core my apples when juicing.

Remove the beet tops from your beets. Remove the tops from the carrots, then cut them into smaller chunks to fit them more easily in your hopper.

Add the ingredients to the hopper in this order: First layer your apples, then add the beets and carrots on top for a smoother juicing process.

Once it's loaded, turn on the juicer and run it until all the ingredients are juiced.

Pour your juice into 16-ounce (480-ml) containers for seven servings. Fill them all the way to the top if storing in the fridge, and leave space in the container if you plan on freezing.

NOTE: You can use Honeycrisp, Pink Lady and Fuji apples as well.

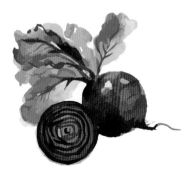

TANGY ABC

Growing up, my mom loved making me juices with tons of red beets. They have many health benefits such as supporting healthy liver function, menstruation and healthy blood flow. I created this juice to help get more red beets in. And if you're not a beet lover, this one is great to try out! The carrots and oranges give this juice a sweet, refreshing balance.

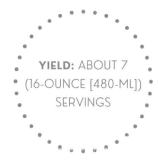

YIELD: ABOUT 7 (16-OUNCE [480-ML]) SERVINGS

• •

GET JUICING!

Wash all your produce and get ready to prep.

Peel the oranges and lemons. Remove the tops from the carrots, then cut them into smaller chunks to fit them more easily in your hopper.

There is no need to peel the apples, but you can core them. Nama suggests coring because apple seeds are known to have toxicity; I prefer to core my apples when juicing.

Remove the beet tops from your beets.

Add the ingredients to the hopper in this order: First layer your oranges and lemons, then add the carrots, apples and beets on top for a smoother juicing process.

Once it's loaded, turn on the juicer and run it until all the ingredients are juiced.

Pour your juice into 16-ounce (480-ml) containers for seven servings. Fill them all the way to the top if storing in the fridge, and leave space in the container if you plan on freezing.

JUICING LINE UP

15 ORANGES

3 LEMONS

6 LB (2.7 KG) CARROTS

4 LARGE APPLES

4 BEETS

• •

NOTE: I like to use Cosmic Crisp apples in this blend. They are a perfect balance of sweetness and tartness. I definitely recommend them!

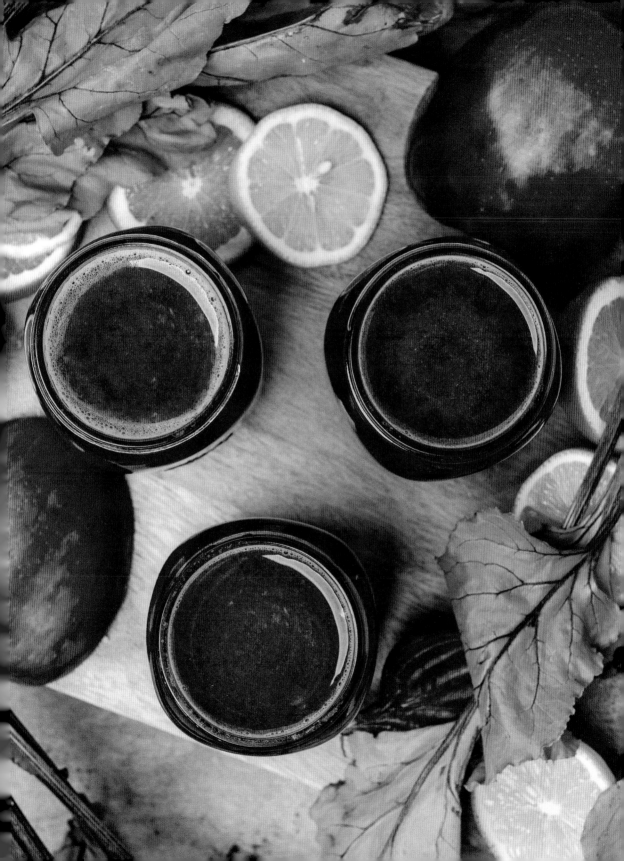

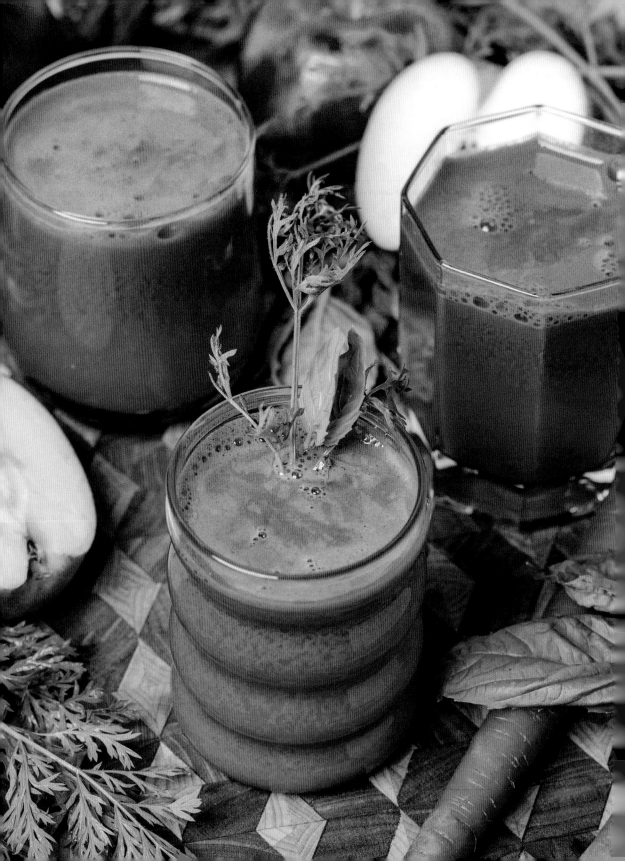

BOOSTING MEDLEY

Basil is up there when it comes to elevating flavor. It's so easy to grow indoors or outdoors, and it saves you money and is always on hand. This juice has antibacterial and anti-inflammatory properties, and it is packed with vitamin C. It also supports eye health and helps protect against UV rays from the sun!

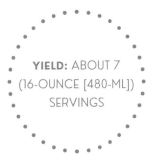

YIELD: ABOUT 7 (16-OUNCE [480-ML]) SERVINGS

GET JUICING!

Wash all your produce and get ready to prep.

Remove the tops from the carrots, then cut them into smaller chunks to fit them more easily in your hopper.

There is no need to peel the apples, but you can core them. Nama suggests coring because apple seeds are known to have toxicity; I prefer to core my apples when juicing.

Add the ingredients to the hopper in this order: First layer your basil, then add the apples and carrots on top for a smoother juicing process.

Once it's loaded, turn on the juicer and run it until all the ingredients are juiced.

Pour your juice into 16-ounce (480-ml) containers for seven servings. Fill them all the way to the top if storing in the fridge, and leave space in the container if you plan on freezing.

NOTE: You can use Honeycrisp, Pink Lady and Fuji apples as well.

JUICING LINE UP

¼ CUP (12 G) BASIL

6 COSMIC CRISP APPLES

10 LB (4.5 KG) CARROTS

TWISTED WATERMELON

Drink this before or after your next workout. This juice is packed with electrolytes and antioxidants. These fruits are known to support muscle recovery, help fight bloating and more! The orange and lime give this watermelon juice combo an incredible citrus twist that I hope you enjoy as much as I do!

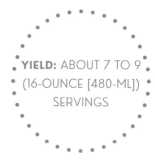

YIELD: ABOUT 7 TO 9 (16-OUNCE [480-ML]) SERVINGS

. . . .

GET JUICING!

Wash all your produce and get ready to prep.

Remove the rind from the watermelon. Cut it into smaller chunks to fit easily in your juicer. Peel the oranges. Use a knife to remove the peels from the limes. Cut the oranges and limes in half.

Add the ingredients to the hopper in any order you like. Layering doesn't matter for this juice, as the ingredients have a similar softness to them.

Once it's loaded, turn on the juicer and run it until all the ingredients are juiced.

Pour your juice into 16-ounce (480-ml) containers for seven servings. Fill them all the way to the top if storing in the fridge, and leave space in the container if you plan on freezing.

JUICING LINE UP

½ OF A WATERMELON

8 ORANGES

4 LIMES

. . . .

NOTES

- You can juice the white part of the watermelon rind if you want to! I prefer to use a seeded watermelon, but you can also use a seedless watermelon for this juice.
- Watermelon has tons of water content; how much juice you get will depend on how juicy yours is.

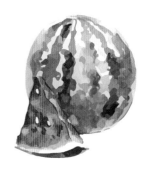

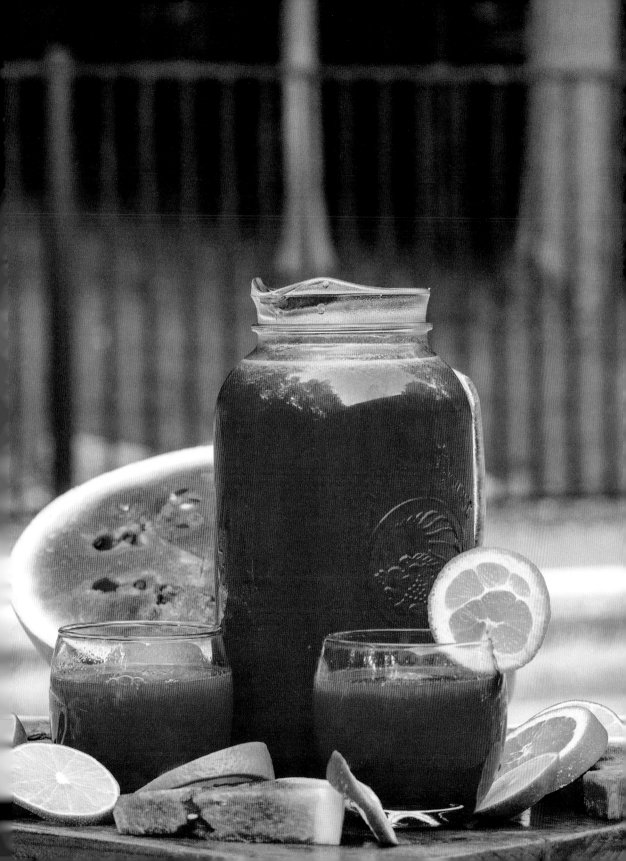

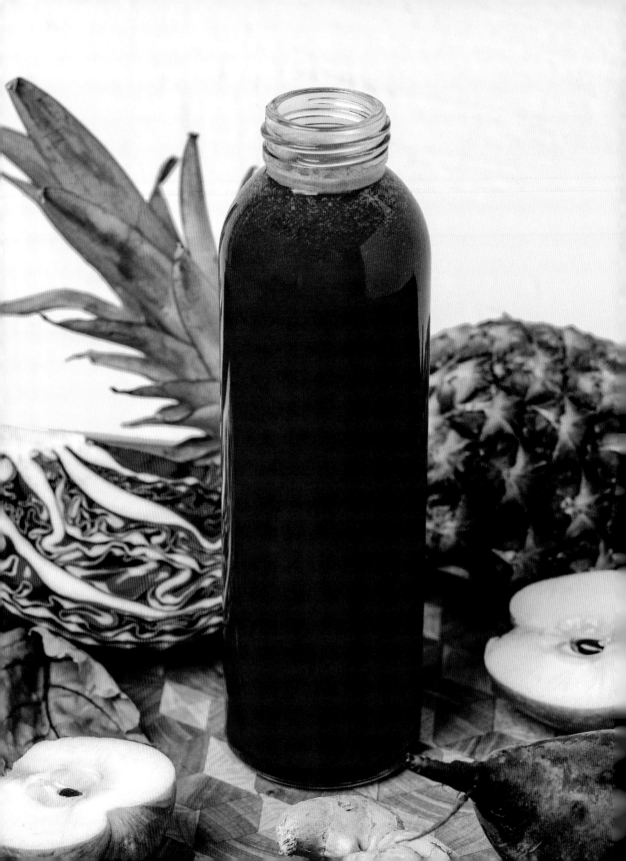

DEEP PURPLE PASSION

Juicing has helped me consume more purple cabbage, which means I get to enjoy all the amazing health benefits that come with it. Cabbage is known for its gut-supporting properties. It also supports your body's natural detoxification, has anticancer properties, helps support hormone balance and more. Adding pineapple gives this the right amount of sweetness. This is one of my favorite purple cabbage combos!

GET JUICING!

Wash all your produce and get ready to prep.

Remove the crown from the pineapples and remove the skins. I don't core my pineapple; I like to keep it because there are many nutrients found in the core. Once you remove the skin from your pineapple, cut it into small chunks.

Remove a few of the outer leaves from the cabbages, including any that are damaged or wilted. Cut it into pieces to fit easily in the hopper.

There is no need to peel the apples, but you can core them. Nama suggests coring because apple seeds are known to have toxicity; I prefer to core my apples when juicing.

I like to peel my ginger with a potato peeler, but you can leave it unpeeled if you prefer. Cut the ginger into smaller pieces for a smoother juicing process.

Remove the tops from your beets.

Add the ingredients to the hopper in this order: First layer your pineapples, then add the cabbages, apples, ginger and beets on top for a smoother juicing process. Once it's loaded, turn on the juicer and run it until all the ingredients are juiced.

Pour your juice into 16-ounce (480-ml) containers for seven servings. Fill them all the way to the top if storing in the fridge, and leave space in the container if you plan on freezing.

JUICING LINE UP

3 PINEAPPLES

1½ CABBAGES

3 APPLES

3 (3-INCH [7.5-CM]) PIECES OF GINGER, OPTIONAL

3 SMALL BEETS

TIP: For easier washing, cut the cabbages in half. I spray them with a veggie wash (page 13), then rinse them.

TROPICAL HARMONY

My mom would always try to get me to eat papaya as a kid, and I just couldn't. The smell and flavor on its own were too much for me. If only she'd had this juice combo! Rather than buying conventional juice filled with syrups and added sugars . . . try this one! It's filled with fruity goodness and it's delicious. Great for sharing, once you make this you'll wonder why you ever bought grocery store juice. It's also packed with vitamin C, immune system–supporting benefits, gut health, anti-inflammatory properties, digestive support and so much more. It's great to freeze as popsicles for kids . . . and adults!

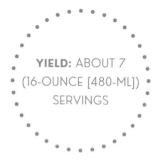

YIELD: ABOUT 7 (16-OUNCE [480-ML]) SERVINGS

JUICING LINE UP

1 PINT (312 G) RASPBERRIES

11 ORANGES

5 LIMES

1 PAPAYA

1 PINEAPPLE

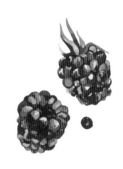

GET JUICING!

Wash all your produce and get ready to prep.

Peel the oranges. Use a knife to remove the peels from the limes, and cut them in half. Peel the papaya and cut it into chunks to fit easily in the hopper.

Remove the crown from the pineapple and remove the skin. I don't core my pineapple; I like to keep it because there are many nutrients found in the core. Once you remove the skin from your pineapple, cut it into small chunks.

Add the ingredients to the hopper in this order: First layer your raspberries, then add the oranges, limes, papaya and pineapple on top for a smoother juicing process. Once it's loaded, turn on the juicer and run it until all the ingredients are juiced.

Pour your juice into 16-ounce (480-ml) containers for seven servings. Fill them all the way to the top if storing in the fridge, and leave space in the container if you plan on freezing.

NOTE: Papaya seeds are known to clear parasites from the intestines. They are edible, but they are bitter and do change the taste of your juice.

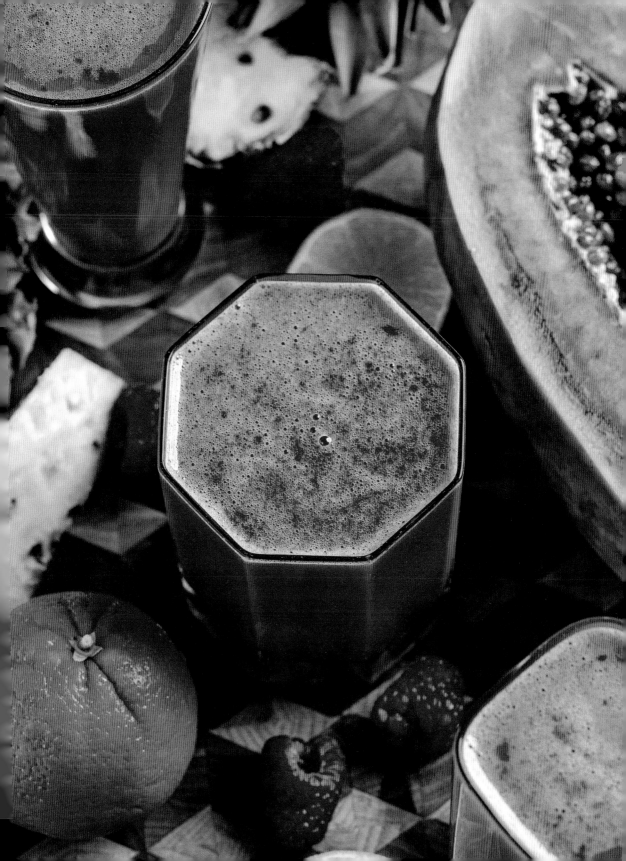

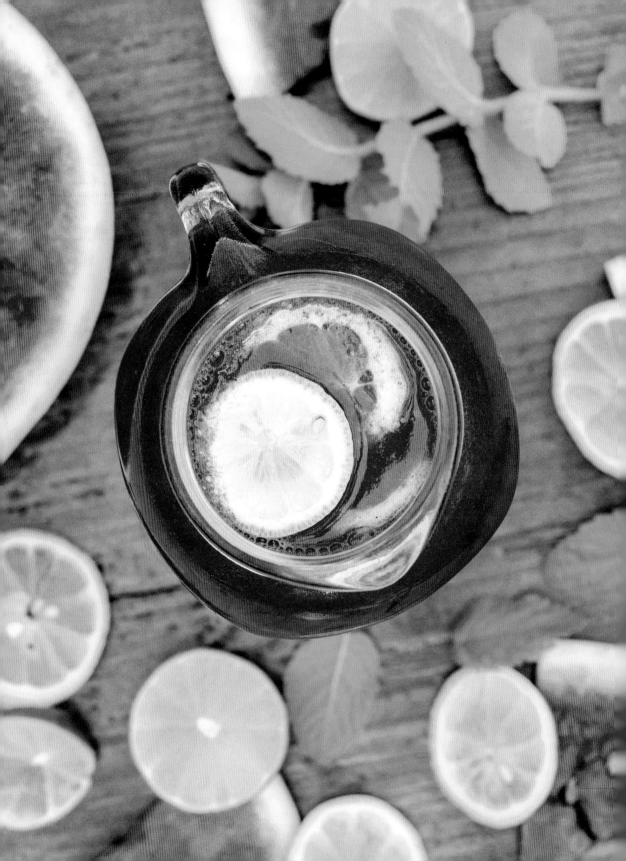

SWEET RECOVERY

Hydration and muscle recovery? Count me in! Watermelon is one of my favorite fruits to juice. It's cost-effective and high in water content, which means more juice and more hydration. It's great before and after a workout to support your muscle recovery, and it helps minimize the potential for cramps after working out. This juice combo is a refreshingly simple way to get electrolytes in and stay hydrated. Feel free to keep this refreshing delicious juice to yourself or share it!

YIELD: ABOUT 7 TO 9 (16-OUNCE [480-ML]) SERVINGS

GET JUICING!

Wash all your produce and get ready to prep.

Remove the green rind from the watermelon. Cut the rest into chunks to fit easily into the hopper. Peel the lemons. Use a knife to remove the peels from the limes. Cut the lemons and the limes in half.

Add the ingredients to the hopper in any order you like. Layering doesn't matter for this juice, as the ingredients have a similar softness to them.

Once it's loaded, turn on the juicer and run it until all the ingredients are juiced.

Pour your juice into 16-ounce (480-ml) containers for seven servings. Fill them all the way to the top if storing in the fridge, and leave space in the container if you plan on freezing.

JUICING LINE UP

1 SEEDLESS WATERMELON

5 LEMONS

4 LIMES

¼ CUP (24 G) MINT, OPTIONAL

NOTES

- You can juice the white part of the watermelon rind if you want to. I usually do!
- Watermelon has tons of water content; sometimes you can get seven to nine 16-ounce (480-ml) servings.

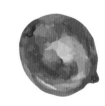

SOOTHING CELERY

Keep it simple with celery juice! Many people's first experience with juicing probably started when they wanted to get their hands on celery juice. It is known for reducing inflammation and improving gut health. It also supports metabolism and the body's natural detoxification. It can be expensive to buy at juice bars . . . and it's so simple and cost-effective to make at home. I like adding lemon to mine for a more refreshing citrus flavor.

GET JUICING!

Wash all your produce and get ready to prep.

Peel the lemons and cut them in half. Cut the celery ribs into quarters for a smoother juicing process.

Add the ingredients to the hopper in this order: First layer your lemons, then add the celery on top for a smoother juicing process.

Once it's loaded, turn on the juicer and run it until all the ingredients are juiced.

Pour your juice into 16-ounce (480-ml) containers for seven servings. Fill them all the way to the top if storing in the fridge, and leave space in the container if you plan on freezing.

NOTE: When I make this recipe, I use organic celery, which means the ribs tend to be smaller than nonorganic. If using nonorganic, use eight or nine.

YIELD: ABOUT 7 (16-OUNCE [480-ML]) SERVINGS

JUICING LINE UP

4 LEMONS

11 RIBS ORGANIC CELERY

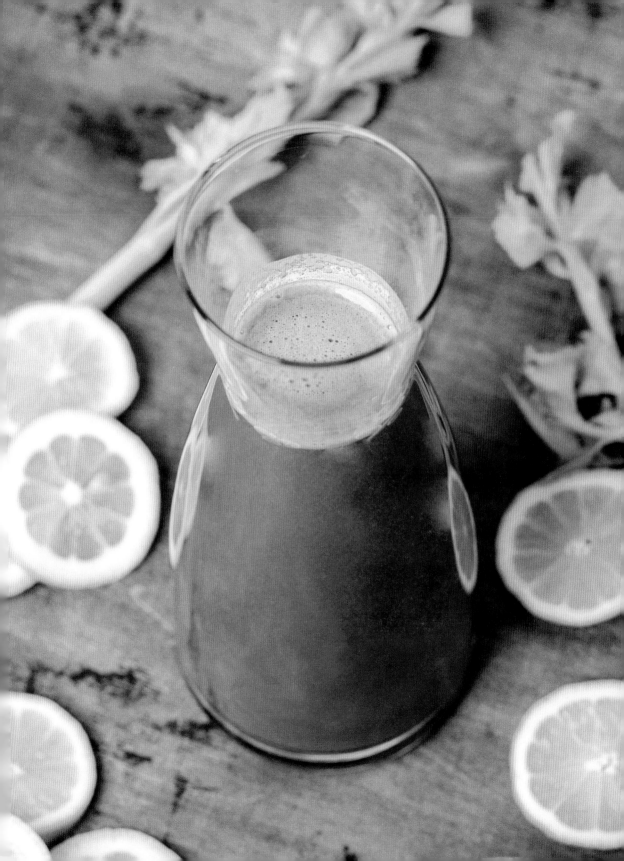

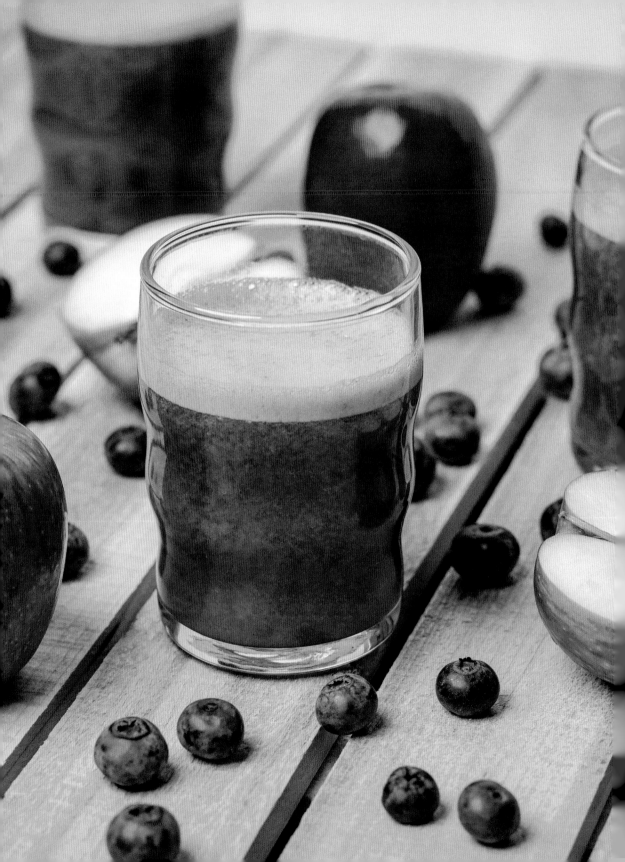

APPLE BLUEBREEZE

If there was one season I could live in year-round, it would be fall. I live in Michigan, and I love watching the leaves change. The air gets crisp and cool, and we take trips to the cider mill for fresh cider. It really doesn't feel like fall until I make my way over and grab some. This cider-inspired juice tides me over during the rest of the year while I wait for fall to come around again. I love adding blueberries to give this combo the brain-supporting properties that blueberries are known for.

YIELD: ABOUT 7 (16-OUNCE [480-ML]) SERVINGS

JUICING LINE UP

2 PINTS (620 G) BLUEBERRIES

12 APPLES

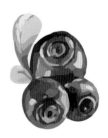

GET JUICING!

Wash all your produce and get ready to prep.

There is no need to peel the apples, but you can core them. Nama suggests coring because apple seeds are known to have toxicity; I prefer to core my apples when juicing.

Add the ingredients to the hopper in this order: First layer your blueberries, then add the apples on top for a smoother juicing process.

Once it's loaded, turn on the juicer and run it until all the ingredients are juiced.

Pour your juice into 16-ounce (480-ml) containers for seven servings. Fill them all the way to the top if storing in the fridge, and leave space in the container if you plan on freezing.

NOTE: Blueberries do give the juice a thicker consistency. Make sure to give it a good shake when ready to consume.

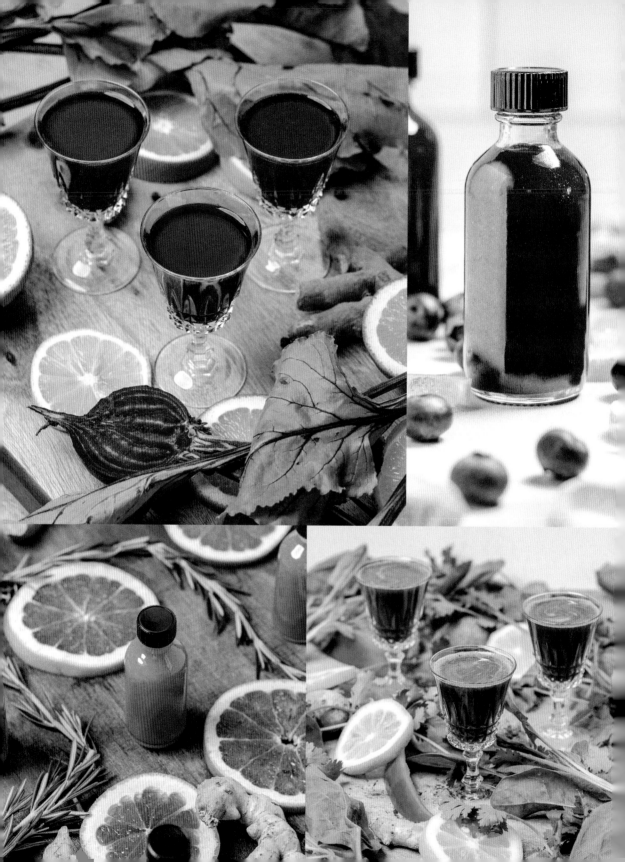

DRINK THE RAINBOW
WELLNESS SHOTS

Wellness shots are a quick way to get essential nutrients in your day-to-day life. Grab one before leaving home, or pack them up for your lunch. Juice shots can ease you into larger servings and give you an opportunity to try out a new-to-you fruit, veggie or combo. Or, if you aren't ready to buy tons of produce for a bigger batch, they are a great way to spend less and still stay consistent with your juicing routine.

These shots give you a spectrum of nutrients found in all the colorful fruits and veggies. They get you closer to eating—well, drinking—the rainbow.

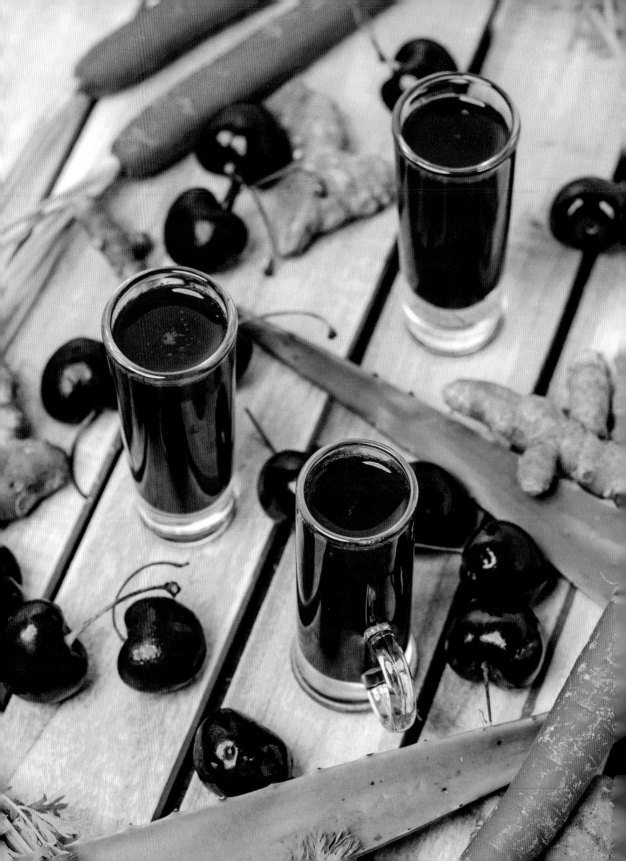

JUICY GLOW

Start your skin care routine on the inside! Aloe is known for its skin repair and topical health benefits. Loaded with carrot, turmeric and cherry, these little wellness shots are packed with antioxidants, mood-boosting properties and wonderful juicy flavor!

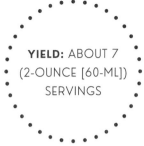

YIELD: ABOUT 7 (2-OUNCE [60-ML]) SERVINGS

GET JUICING!

Wash all your produce and get ready to prep.

Remove the pits and stems from the cherries. Remove the top from the carrot, then cut it into smaller chunks to fit it more easily in your hopper.

Add the cherries, turmeric and aloe gel to the hopper. Once it's loaded, turn on the juicer and run it until all the ingredients are juiced.

Add the carrot and rerun the pulp through the juicer.

Stir the black pepper into the juice. Pour the juice into seven 2-ounce (60-ml) containers.

JUICING LINE UP

30 CHERRIES

2 (3-INCH [7.5-CM]) PIECES OF TURMERIC

1 CUP (240 ML) ALOE GEL

1 LARGE CARROT

½ TSP BLACK PEPPER

TIPS

- Juicing the carrot last will help push out any pulp that is stuck in your juicer.
- The gel might be hard to get into the small-mouthed shot glasses; try a wider-mouthed shot glass for easy pouring.

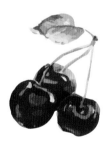

GET UP AND GO

Pineapple, beet and ginger are energizers, and they make a surprisingly sweet combo! Ginger is wonderful first thing in the morning, so these wellness shots make a good addition to your next rotation. Who doesn't want some energy, an iron boost and healthy blood flow?

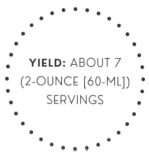

YIELD: ABOUT 7 (2-OUNCE [60-ML]) SERVINGS

GET JUICING!

Wash all your produce and get ready to prep.

Remove the crown from the pineapple and remove the skin. I don't core my pineapple; I like to keep it because there are many nutrients found in the core. Once you remove the skin from your pineapple, cut it into small chunks.

Remove the tops from your beets. I like to peel my ginger with a potato peeler, but you can leave it unpeeled if you prefer. Cut the ginger into smaller pieces for a smoother juicing process.

Add the ingredients to the hopper in this order: First layer your pineapple, then add the beets and ginger on top for a smoother juicing process.

Once it's loaded, turn on the juicer and run it until all the ingredients are juiced.

Pour the juice into seven 2-ounce (60-ml) shot glasses.

NOTE: If the beets have leaves, they can be juiced as well. Keep in mind they do change the taste of your wellness shots.

JUICING LINE UP

¼ OF A PINEAPPLE

2 MEDIUM RED BEETS

1 (4-INCH [10-CM]) PIECE OF GINGER

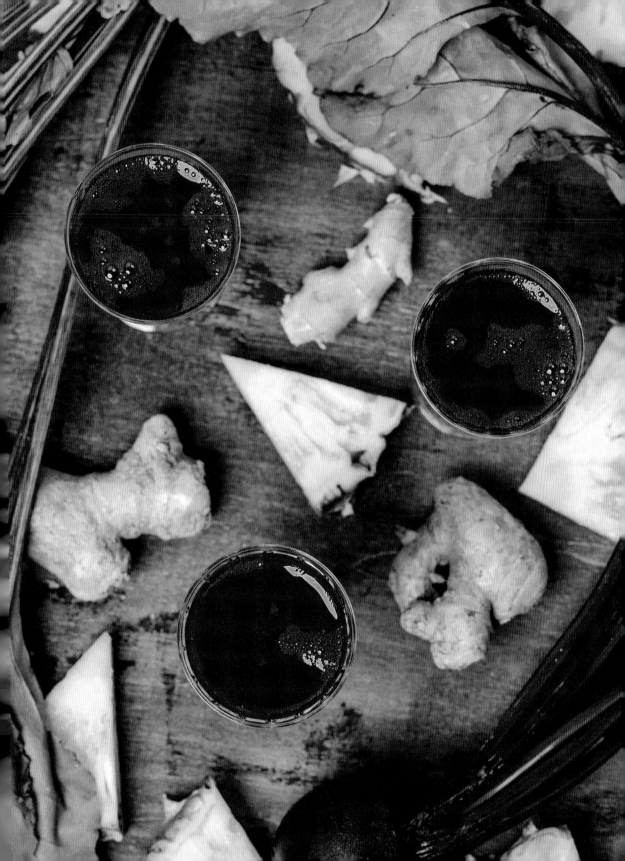

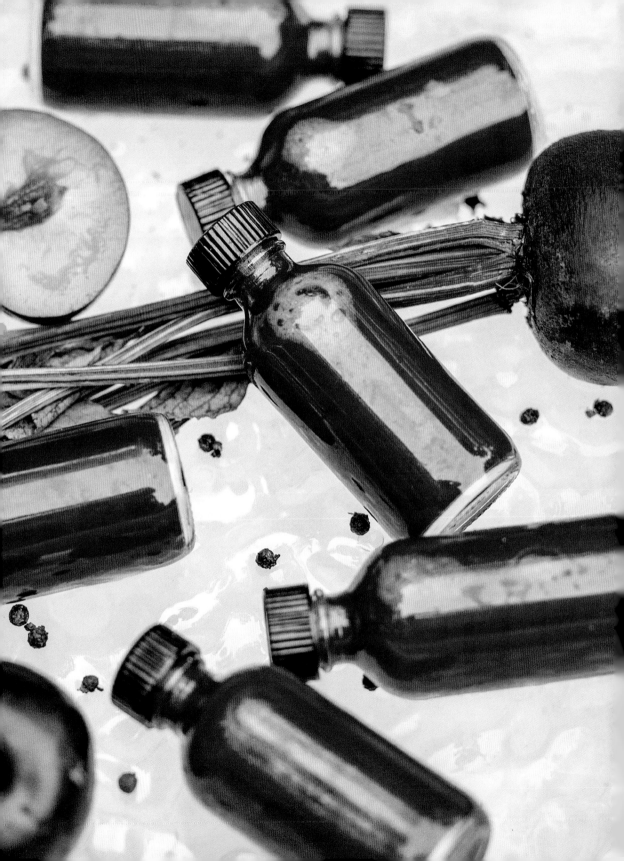

FLOWING PLUM WELLNESS SHOT

This wellness shot is a treat with plums and strawberries shining through. This is a great one to help get the digestive support you need and to help support healthy blood flow. It's a good switch-up from the tangier wellness shots.

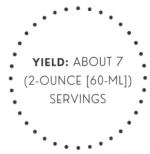

YIELD: ABOUT 7 (2-OUNCE [60-ML]) SERVINGS

. . . .

GET JUICING!

Wash all your produce and get ready to prep.

Remove the pits and stems from the plums. Remove the tops from the beet.

Add the ingredients to the hopper in this order: First layer your plums and strawberries, then add the turmeric and beet on top for a smoother juicing process.

Once it's loaded, turn on the juicer and run it until all the ingredients are juiced.

Stir the black pepper into the juice. Pour the juice into seven 2-ounce (60-ml) containers.

JUICING LINE UP

3 PLUMS

7 STRAWBERRIES

2 (3-INCH [7.5-CM]) PIECES OF TURMERIC

1 MEDIUM BEET

½ TSP BLACK PEPPER

. . . .

TIPS

- When choosing plums, the darker the plums, the sweeter they are.
- Black pepper helps with turmeric absorption.

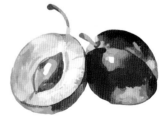

GOLDEN HOUR WELLNESS SHOT

I posted this on social media and it blew up! People loved it, so I have to share it here as well. Skip the coffee and try these small-but-powerful energy boosters! These are great on the go and when you need a dose of vitamins and anti-inflammatory properties that aid your digestion. This recipe will make you think twice about buying wellness shots at the store . . . they're that good.

• •

GET JUICING!
Wash all your produce and get ready to prep.

Peel the oranges, and cut them in half. Use a knife to remove the peel from the lime.

I like to peel my ginger with a potato peeler, but you can leave it unpeeled if you prefer. Cut the ginger into smaller pieces for a smoother juicing process.

Remove the crown from the pineapple and remove the skin. I don't core my pineapple; I like to keep it because there are many nutrients found in the core. Once you remove the skin from your pineapple, cut it into small chunks.

Add the ingredients to the hopper in this order: First layer the oranges, then add the lime, turmeric, ginger and pineapple on top for a smoother juicing process.

Once it's loaded, turn on the juicer and run it until all the ingredients are juiced.

Stir the black pepper into the juice. Pour the juice into six 2-ounce (60-ml) shot glasses.

YIELD: ABOUT 6 (2-OUNCE [60-ML]) SERVINGS

JUICING LINE UP

2 ORANGES

½ OF A LIME

1 (5-INCH [13-CM]) PIECE OF TURMERIC

1 (4-INCH [10-CM]) PIECE OF GINGER

½ OF A PINEAPPLE

½ TSP BLACK PEPPER

• • • • • • • • • • • •

TIP: Make sure your pineapple isn't overripe to avoid it becoming mush in your hopper. Overripe pineapples can also cause more foam in juice than you would expect. Make sure your pineapple is still slightly green.

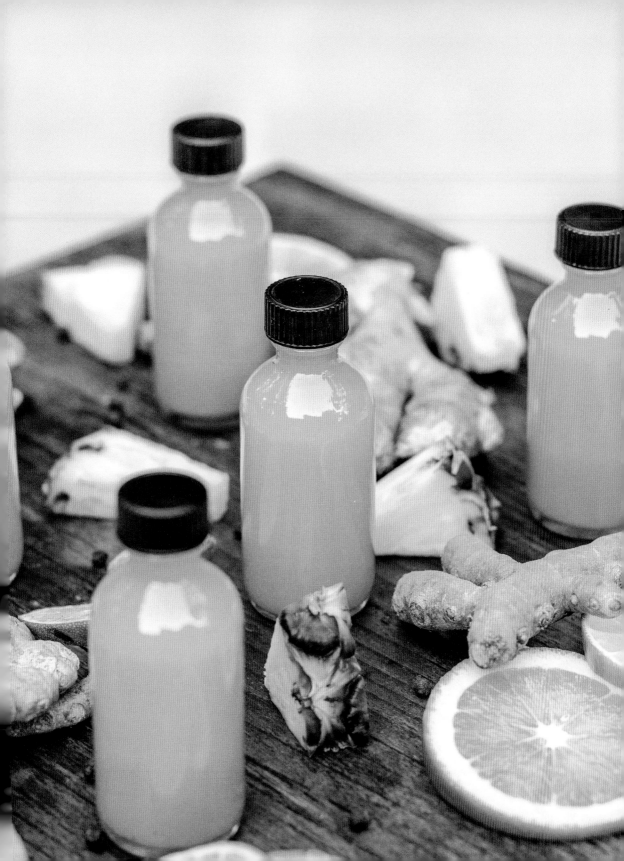

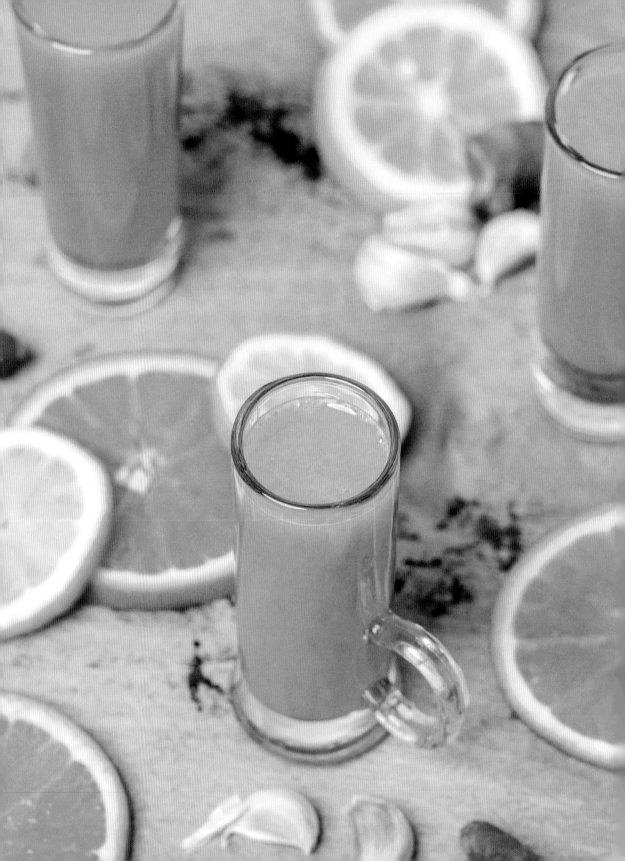

TURMERIC DEFENSE SHOT

Growing up, if I had a scratchy throat, there was a cold going around or I was feeling sick, my parents always had me take minced garlic with water or lime juice and honey mixed together. I would take it morning and night to help fight whatever sickness was trying to come my way— and it worked. Garlic is known for its medicinal properties, and as I've gotten older, I've found ways to make this easy and tasty to drink. If you're feeling under the weather or there's a cold going around, take one of these for that added immune system support!

. . . .

GET JUICING!

Wash all your produce and get ready to prep.

Peel the oranges and lemon. Remove the skin from the garlic clove.

Add the ingredients to the hopper in any order you like. Layering doesn't matter for this, as it's a smaller batch.

Once it's loaded, turn on the juicer and run it until all the ingredients are juiced.

Stir the black pepper into the juice (if using). Pour the juice into seven 2-ounce (60-ml) shot glasses.

. . . .

TIP: If you aren't a fan of garlic, gradually add it into this shot little by little until you get used to the taste.

YIELD: ABOUT 7 (2-OUNCE [60-ML]) SERVINGS

JUICING LINE UP

4 ORANGES

1 LEMON

2 CLOVES GARLIC

2 (3-INCH [7.5-CM]) PIECES OF TURMERIC

½ TSP BLACK PEPPER, OPTIONAL

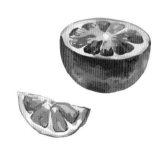

GARDEN GREENS SHOT

Grow these ingredients in your garden or on your patio, and support your body's natural detoxification with this easy juice. If you're feeling sleepy, take a shot of this. Trust me: It will wake you up! This is one of my favorite shots to take for a quick morning boost, and it also packs in some great health benefits to start the day.

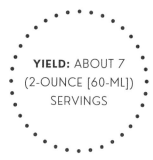

YIELD: ABOUT 7 (2-OUNCE [60-ML]) SERVINGS

GET JUICING!

Wash your leafy greens and other produce, and get ready to prep.

Remove any wilted or slimy cilantro leaves. Peel the lemons and cut them in half. Cut the bell pepper in half and remove the seeds.

I like to peel my ginger with a potato peeler, but you can leave it unpeeled if you prefer. Cut the ginger into smaller pieces for a smoother juicing process.

Add the ingredients to the hopper in this order: First layer your leafy greens, then add the lemons, bell pepper and ginger on top for a smoother juicing process.

Once it's loaded, turn on the juicer and run it until all the ingredients are juiced.

Pour the juice into seven 2-ounce (60-ml) shot glasses.

JUICING LINE UP

4 PACKED CUPS (140 G) SPINACH

1 BUNCH CILANTRO

2 LEMONS

1 BELL PEPPER

1 (5-INCH [13-CM]) PIECE OF GINGER

TIP: Remove the seeds from the bell pepper to give the juice a less peppery taste.

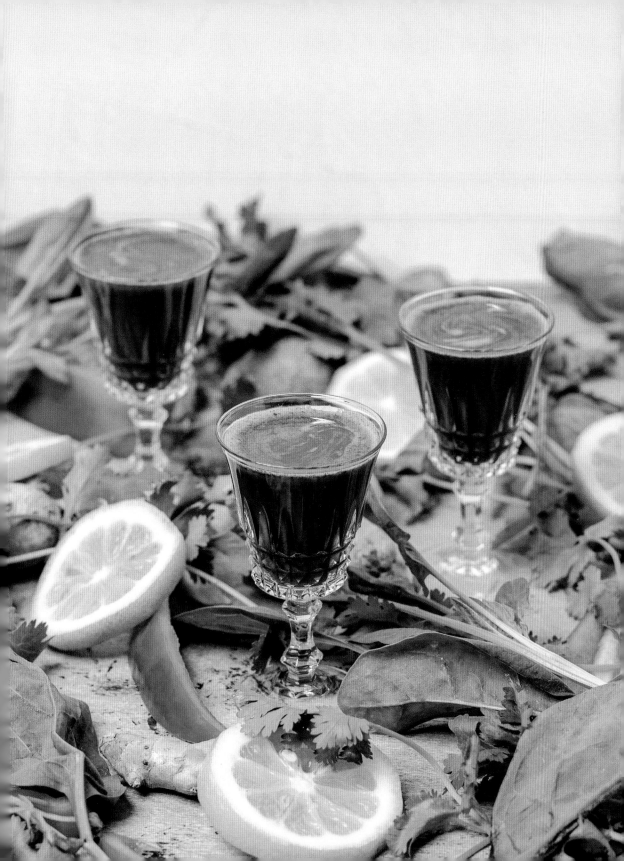

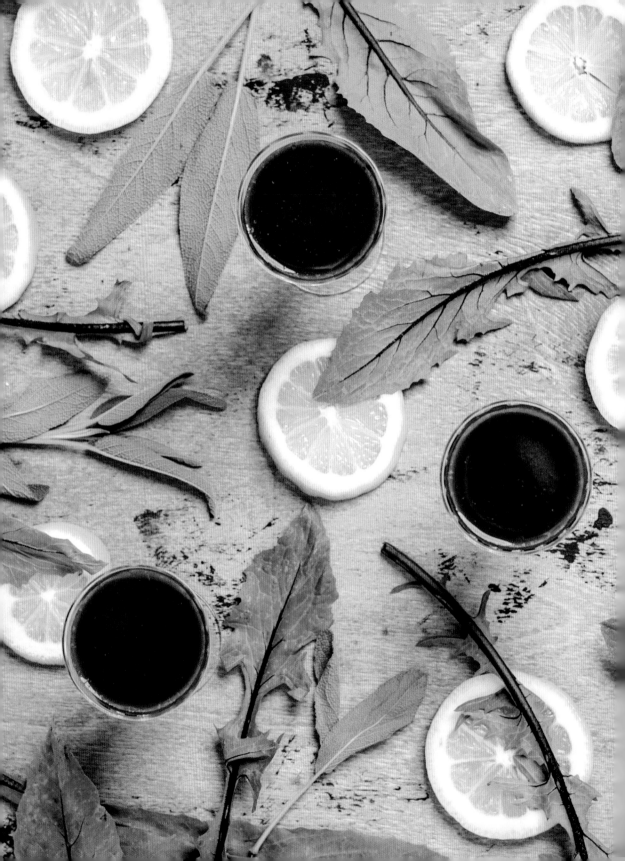

BRAIN BOOST GREENS SHOT

Don't let brain fog get the best of you! Sage is known to help support brain function, and dandelion greens are known to help support natural liver detoxification and the digestive system. Keep your body and mind nourished!

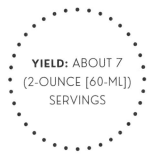

YIELD: ABOUT 7 (2-OUNCE [60-ML]) SERVINGS

• •

GET JUICING!

Wash all your produce and get ready to prep.

Remove any wilted or slimy leaves from the dandelion greens. Peel the lemons.

Add the ingredients to the hopper in any order you like. Layering doesn't matter for this, as it's a smaller batch.

Once it's loaded, turn on the juicer and run it until all the ingredients are juiced.

Pour the juice into seven 2-ounce (60-ml) shot glasses.

JUICING LINE UP

1 BUNCH DANDELION GREENS (AROUND 10 OZ [283 G])

3 LEMONS

3 SPRIGS SAGE

• •

TIP: You can chop the dandelion greens for a smoother juicing process.

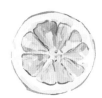

BEET-IFUL

Are you looking for a wellness shot that helps support your body's natural detoxification, healthy liver function, digestion and more? I've got the wellness shot for you. I'm not a red beet type of person, but believe me when I tell you that nothing "beets" this delicious wellness shot. Tangy, citrusy and slightly earthy, these have more of a sweet, beet-y taste. The balance of the black pepper and turmeric gives these an amazing flavor, and I know you'll be making them regularly.

. . . .

GET JUICING!

Wash all your produce and get ready to prep.

Peel your oranges and lemon. Remove the tops of your beets and cut them in half.

Add the ingredients to the hopper in this order: First layer your oranges, then add the lemon, turmeric and beets on top for a smoother juicing process.

Once it's loaded, turn on the juicer and run it until all the ingredients are juiced.

Stir the black pepper into the juice. Pour the juice into seven 2-ounce (60-ml) shot glasses.

. . . .

TIP: If you want to make the most of your beets, you can also juice the stems and leafy greens.

YIELD: ABOUT 7
(2-OUNCE [60-ML])
SERVINGS

JUICING LINE UP

3 ORANGES

1 LEMON

2 (3-INCH [7.5-CM])
PIECES OF TURMERIC

2 RED BEETS

½ TSP BLACK PEPPER

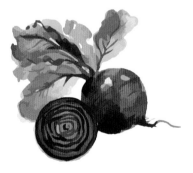

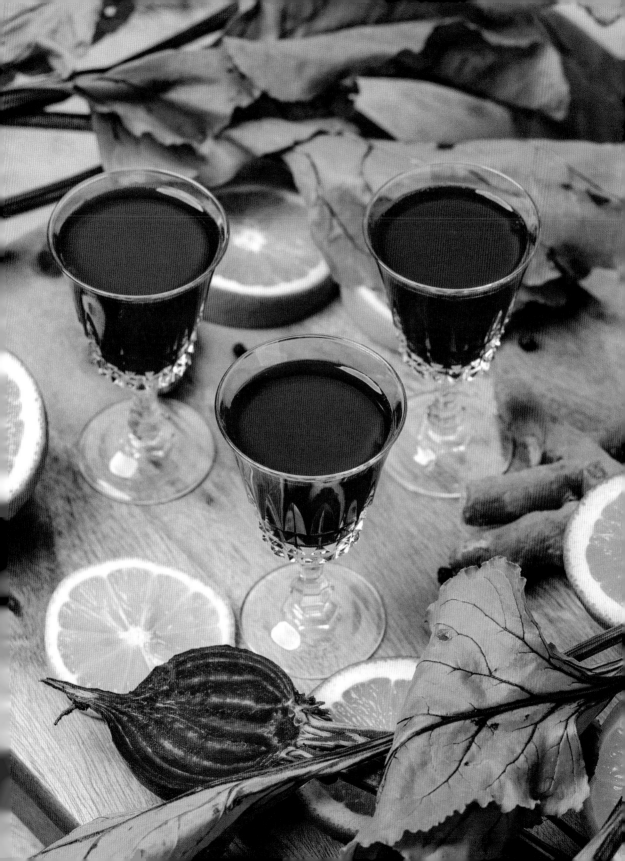

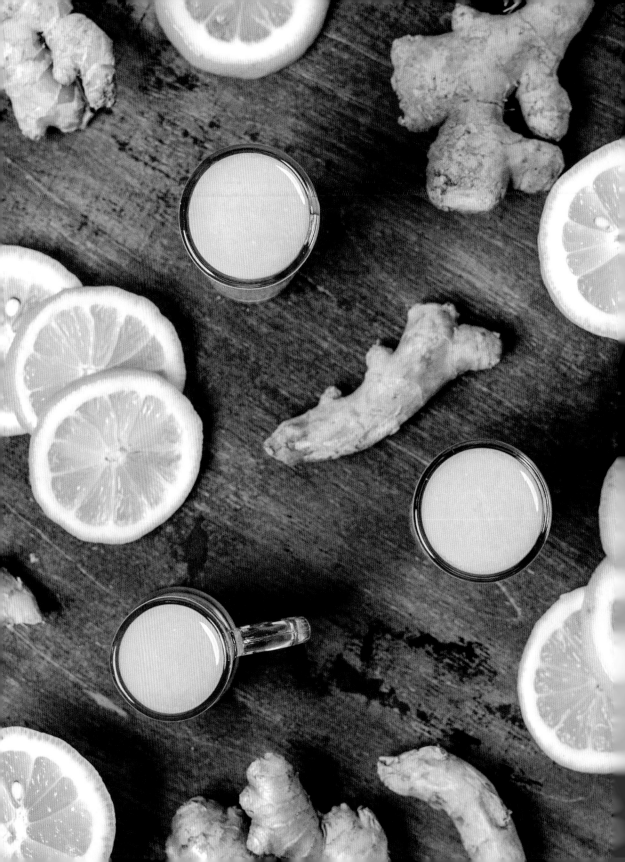

GINGER ZING

This is probably one of the easiest, most cost-effective wellness shots that you can make. The ingredients help alleviate nausea and stomach issues, provide digestive support and reduce inflammation. I almost always have lemons and ginger on hand, which makes this a convenient wellness shot to make during the week when I am low on other produce.

YIELD: ABOUT 7 (2-OUNCE [60-ML]) SERVINGS

• •

GET JUICING!

Wash all your produce and get ready to prep.

Peel the lemons. I like to peel my ginger with a potato peeler, but you can leave it unpeeled if you prefer. Cut the ginger into smaller pieces for a smoother juicing process.

Add the ingredients to the hopper in any order you like. Layering doesn't matter for this, as it's a smaller batch.

Once it's loaded, turn on the juicer and run it until all the ingredients are juiced.

Pour the mixture into seven 2-ounce (60-ml) shot glasses.

JUICING LINE UP

7 SMALL LEMONS

3 (3-INCH [7.5-CM]) PIECES OF GINGER

• •

TIP: If you don't plan on drinking these within 72 hours, leave room in the shot glasses and freeze them (see page 88).

ZESTY FIGHTER

Get your immune system ready to fight cold season. This wellness shot is refreshingly good, and it's packed with vitamin C as well as antiviral, antibacterial and antifungal properties. It's refreshing, and you can definitely feel the ginger's spice! Please note grapefruit can affect certain medications; if you're on medication, talk to your doctor before consuming grapefruit.

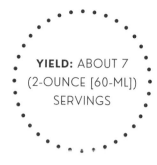

YIELD: ABOUT 7 (2-OUNCE [60-ML]) SERVINGS

JUICING LINE UP

4 GRAPEFRUITS

3 (3-INCH [7.5-CM]) PIECES OF GINGER

2 SPRIGS ROSEMARY

GET JUICING!

Wash all your produce and get ready to prep.

Peel the grapefruits. I like to peel my ginger with a potato peeler, but you can leave it unpeeled if you prefer. Cut the ginger into smaller pieces for a smoother juicing process.

Add the ingredients to the hopper in any order you like. Layering doesn't matter for this, as it's a smaller batch.

Once it's loaded, turn on the juicer and run it until all the ingredients are juiced.

Pour the juice into seven 2-ounce (60-ml) shot glasses.

NOTE: Add in rosemary as a whole sprig. You don't have to only use the leaves.

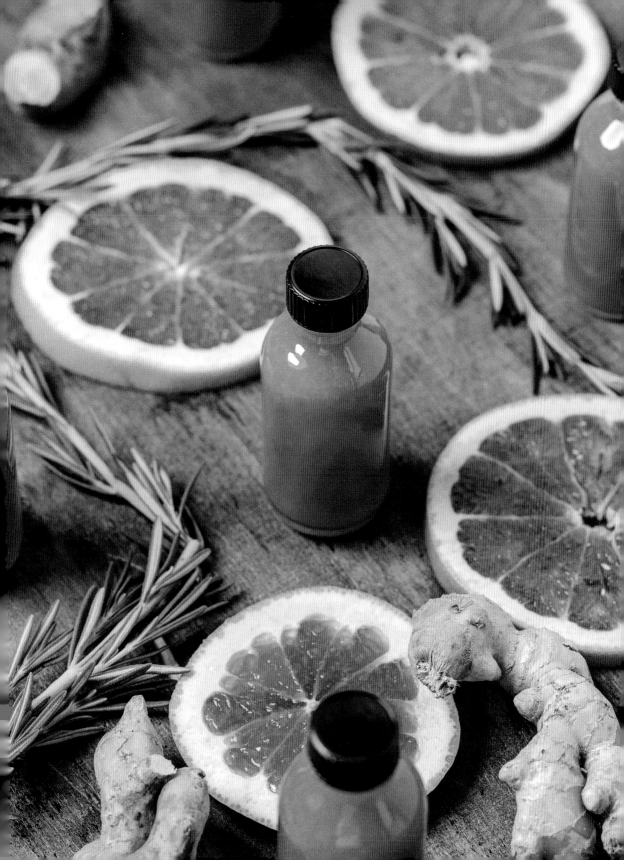

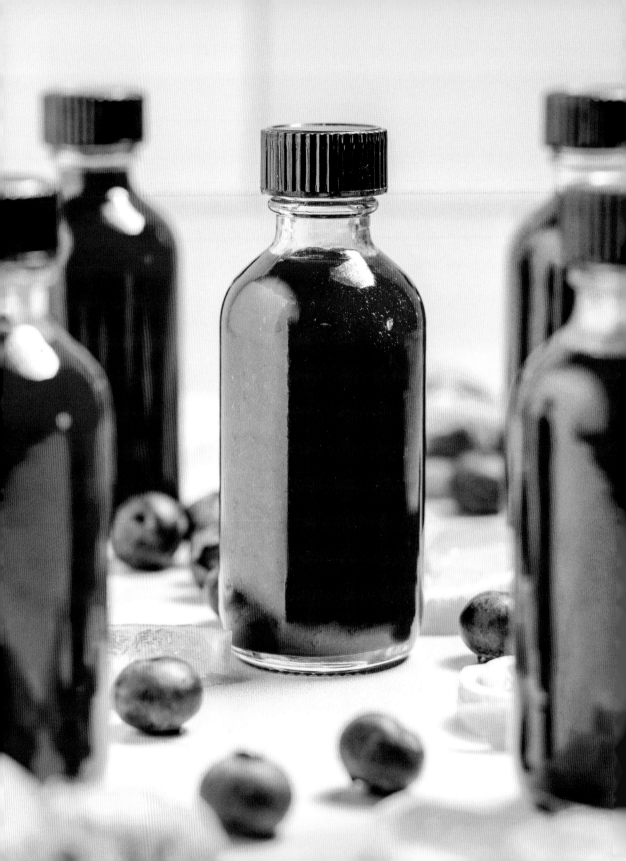

PACKED BERRY

Maintaining healthy brain function is vital, and blueberries are packed with antioxidants that support your brain's health. There's a lot going on in our day-to-day lives. On those days when you are using extra brainpower, make sure that you are equipped with the wellness shot you need. Stay sharp!

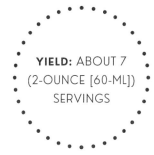

YIELD: ABOUT 7 (2-OUNCE [60-ML]) SERVINGS

GET JUICING!

Wash all your produce and get ready to prep.

Peel the lemons.

Add the ingredients to the hopper in any order you like. Layering doesn't matter for this, as it's a smaller batch.

Once it's loaded, turn on the juicer and run it until all the ingredients are juiced.

Stir the black pepper (if using) into the juice. Pour the juice into seven 2-ounce (60-ml) shot glasses.

JUICING LINE UP

2 LEMONS

1 PINT (310 G) BLUEBERRIES

2 (3-INCH [7.5-CM]) PIECES OF TURMERIC

¼–½ TSP BLACK PEPPER, OPTIONAL

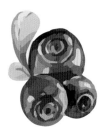

TIPS

- Adding ¼ to ½ teaspoon of black pepper will help with turmeric absorption.
- Keep in mind that blueberries create a thicker juice.

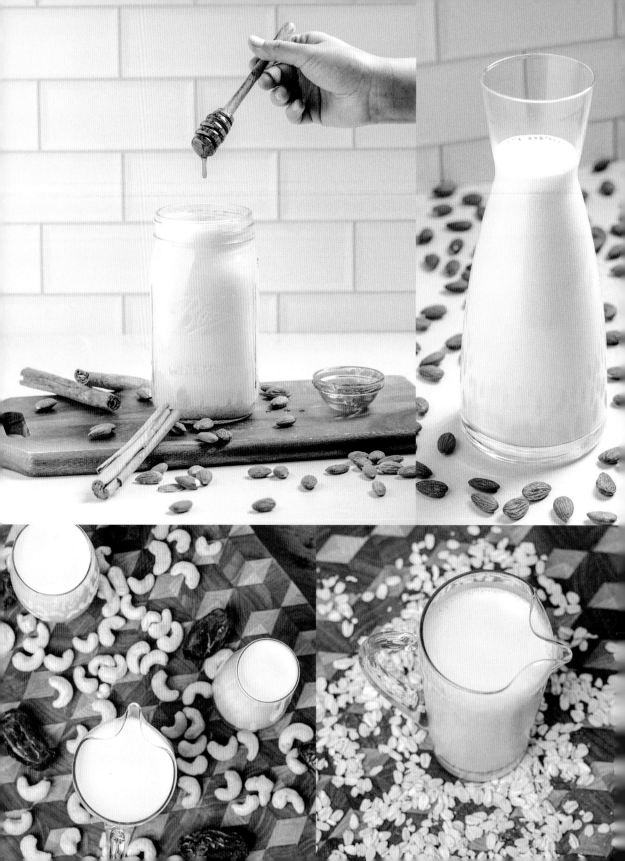

NO DAIRY?
NO PROBLEM!

Grocery store plant-based milks can be expensive, and most include extra ingredients and additives. I love plant-based milk, and I want to know what's in my milk. That is what led me to make my own. And it's so simple to make in your Nama. I didn't realize it until I tried for myself! It only takes a few minutes.

Once you make your own, it's hard to go back to store-bought milk. Homemade is simple and cost-effective, and it preserves the natural nutrients that can be lost through processing. Add these milks to your favorite recipes, smoothies, cereal and more. Once you make and taste your own plant-based milk, you won't want anything else.

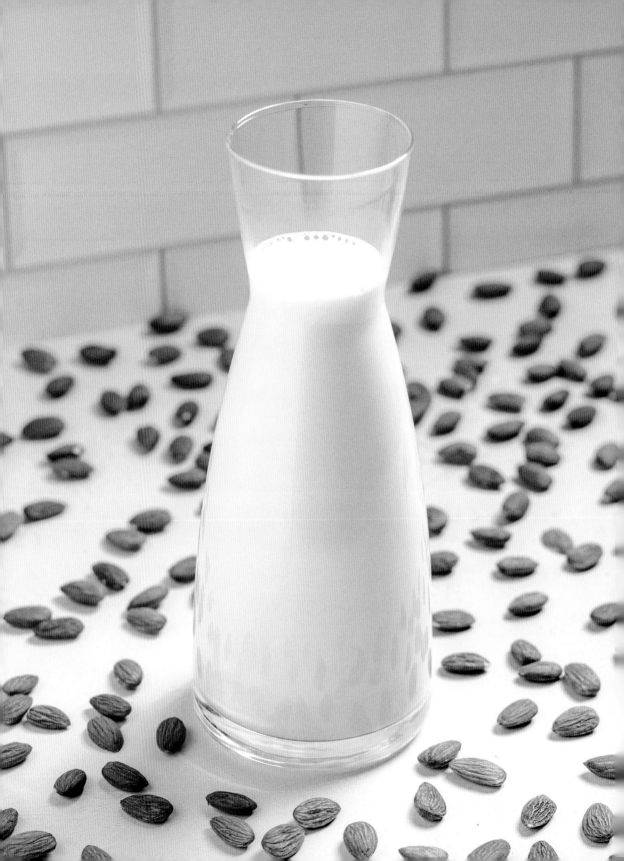

VANILLA ALMOND MILK

People often ask me, "What does homemade almond milk taste like?" I always tell them it's tasty and light, and it's what *real* almond milk should taste like . . . almondy. I like simple almond milk. We go through this pretty quickly in our home so an extra batch always makes sense. Add a pinch of salt to have it last up to five days; it's usually gone by day three for us. This milk is packed with nutrients, healthy fats and vitamin E, which is a powerful antioxidant. Add this to your coffee and favorite recipes. Or if you're like me, drink a small glass before bed to help support better sleep.

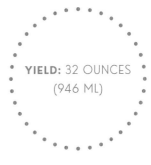

YIELD: 32 OUNCES (946 ML)

JUICING LINE UP

1½ CUPS (218 G) RAW ALMONDS

¼ TSP VANILLA EXTRACT

PINCH OF SALT

GET JUICING!

Add the almonds to a bowl with enough water to cover them, and soak them overnight.

Drain and rinse your soaked almonds. Use a strainer to make it easier. Add 4 cups (946 ml) of fresh cold water to the bowl with your soaked almonds.

Stir the almonds, water and vanilla together. Turn on the juicer and slowly add the mixture to the hopper through the small opening of the lid until all the mixture has been run through.

Pour your milk into a 32-ounce (946-ml) mason jar. With a pinch of salt, the milk keeps in the fridge for 3 to 5 days.

TIP: Make sure you soak your almonds. This makes a nice creamy almond milk and prevents damage to your juicer.

SWEET DREAMS CINNAMON-HONEY ALMOND MILK

Some days I have a lot on my mind, and those thoughts and ideas want to carry into the night and keep me up. Unwind with me and support a good quality of sleep with this heavenly treat. I find this blend comforting and soothing with its naturally occurring melatonin and magnesium to help create a restful night. Sweet dreams!

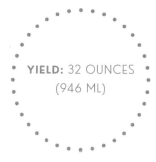

YIELD: 32 OUNCES (946 ML)

JUICING LINE UP

1½ CUPS (218 G) RAW ALMONDS

1½ TSP CINNAMON

¼ TSP VANILLA EXTRACT

1 TBSP (15 ML) HONEY

PINCH OF SALT

GET JUICING!

Add the almonds to a bowl with enough water to cover them, and soak them overnight.

Drain and rinse your soaked almonds. Use a strainer to make it easier. Add 4 cups (946 ml) of fresh cold water to the bowl with your soaked almonds.

Stir the almonds, water, cinnamon and vanilla to combine.

Turn on the juicer and slowly add the mixture to the hopper through the small opening of the lid until all the mixture has been run through.

Pour your milk into a 32-ounce (946-ml) mason jar, and stir in the honey. With a pinch of salt, the milk keeps in the fridge for 3 to 5 days.

TIPS

- Make sure you soak your almonds. This makes a nice creamy almond milk and prevents damage to your juicer.
- I like to use filtered water, as it has a better taste in my opinion.

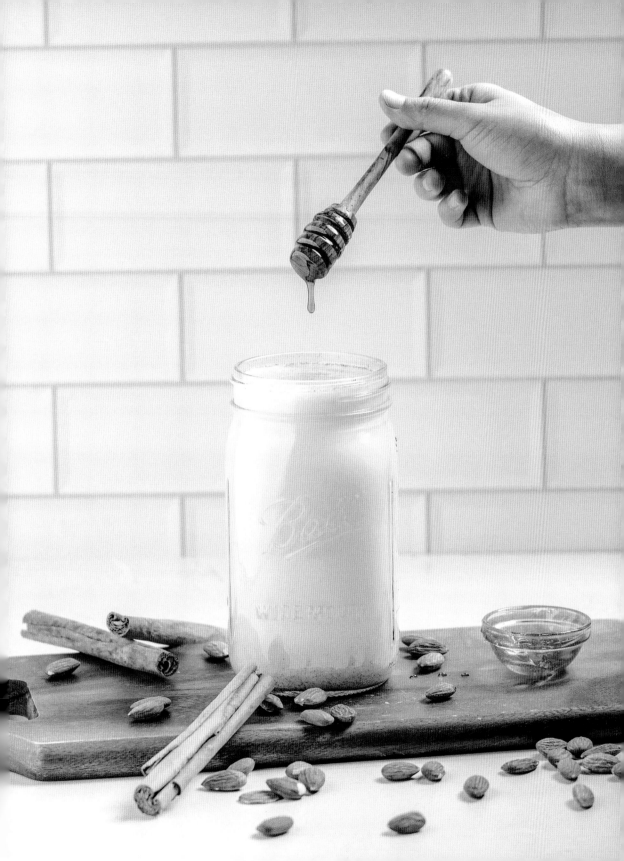

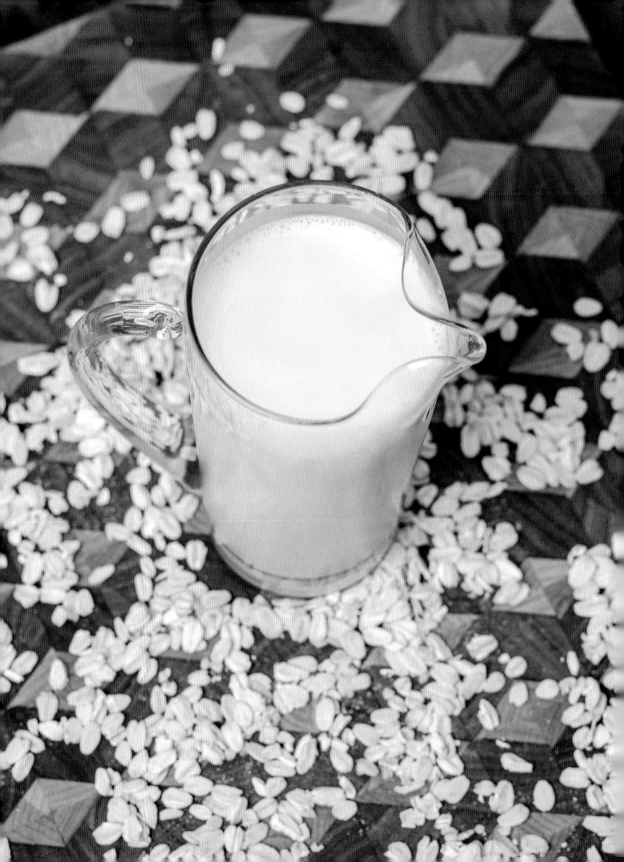

IT'S TWO SIMPLE OAT MILK

I love anything oat! So it's no surprise that I think oat milk is the best-tasting plant-based milk of them all. It's smooth and refreshing. It also doesn't change the flavor drastically when added to your favorite recipes or drinks that need a splash of milk. It has a naturally subtle sweet taste to it and doesn't need any added sweeteners. It's my husband's favorite to add to his morning coffee.

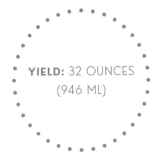

YIELD: 32 OUNCES
(946 ML)

GET JUICING!

Add your oats to a bowl and cover them in cold water. Soak them for 2 hours.

Drain the water and use a strainer to quickly rinse your oats. Once strained, pour 4 cups (946-ml) of fresh cold water into the bowl and add the oats. Stir to combine.

Slowly add the mixture to the hopper through the small opening at the top of the lid until all the mixture has been run through.

Pour your milk into a 32-ounce (946-ml) mason jar. With a pinch of salt, the milk keeps in the fridge for 3 to 5 days.

JUICING LINE UP

1½ CUPS (144 G) OATS

PINCH OF SALT

NOTE: Make sure to use cold water and let the oats soak for the full 2 hours. The cold water keeps the oat milk from becoming slimy and helps the mixture run through the juicer easily.

CASHMOO MILK

If you're looking for creamier milk with less of a nutty taste, try this cashew milk recipe! Packed with nutrients and healthy fats, this is a great milk to make and add to your rotation of plant-based milk.

YIELD: 32 OUNCES (946 ML)

GET JUICING!

Add the cashews and dates to a bowl with enough water to cover them, and soak them overnight.

Drain and rinse your soaked cashews and dates. Use a strainer to make it easier. Add 4 cups (946 ml) of fresh cold water to the bowl with your cashews and dates.

Slowly add the mixture through the small opening at the top of the lid until all the mixture has been run through.

Pour your milk into a 32-ounce (946-ml) mason jar. With a pinch of salt, the milk keeps in the fridge for 3 to 5 days.

JUICING LINE UP

1½ CUPS (205 G) RAW CASHEWS

3 PITTED DATES

PINCH OF SALT

TIPS

- If you want a creamier cashew milk, add more cashews.
- I like to use filtered water, as it has a better flavor in my opinion.

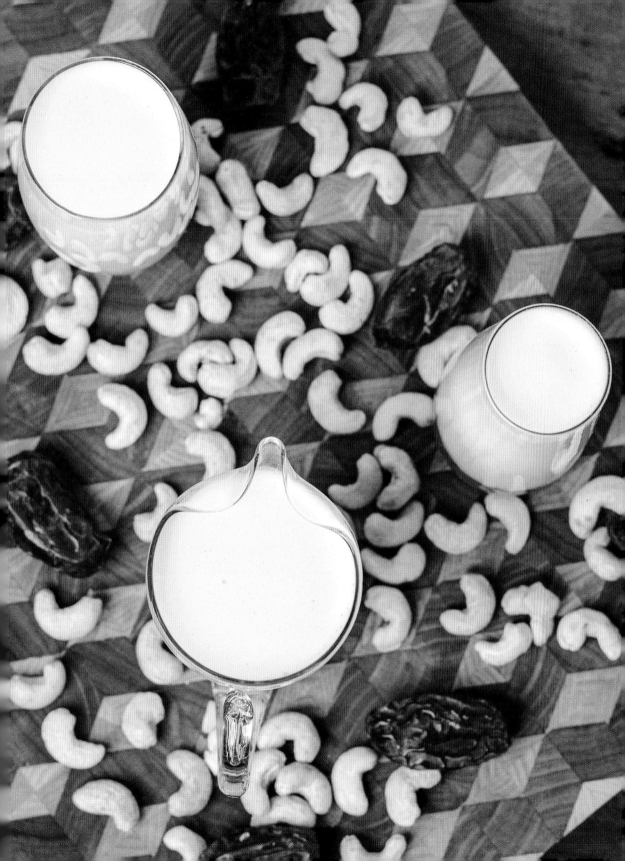

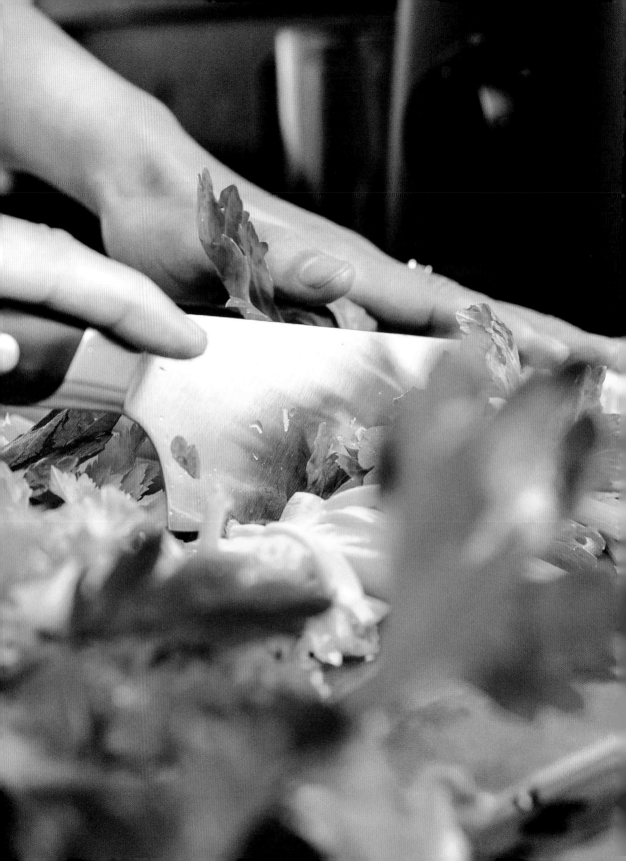

ACKNOWLEDGMENTS

First I want to thank God, for His blessings and opportunities throughout this season in my life.

Thank you to my husband, Jeremy Shane, for being my constant support, love and recipe taste tester. Thank you for always believing in me and cheering me on. I truly could not have done it without you. And of course, thank you for being an incredible photographer and bringing my vision to life. (Yes, he took the photos.)

Thank you to my parents, Jorge and Veronica Velasco, and my parents-in-law, John and Brenda Shane, for your words of encouragement and confidence in me throughout the process.

Thank you to my sisters Jennifer and Jocelyn Velasco for always providing laughs when I need them and for believing in me.

Thank you to my family and friends who have been cheering me on since Day 1!

Thank you to Marissa Giambelluca and the entire team at Page Street Publishing for believing in me and my recipes and for your guidance throughout the whole process.

Thank you to the Nama Team for always cheering me on throughout the process and also for having the best juicer on the market.

Thank you to *everyone* who has been supporting my page and content these past couple of years. This wouldn't be possible without you! I am still in disbelief that I have an incredible community from all over cheering me on and supporting my juice recipes! I love you guys!

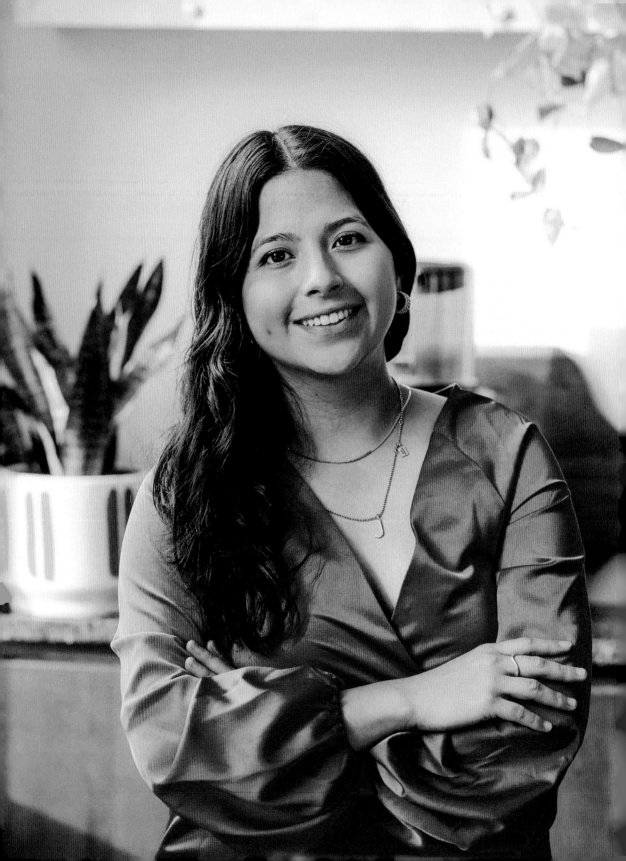

ABOUT THE AUTHOR

Jeanette Velasco Shane is the creator of Juicy Juicing J, a popular page on social media that was launched in the spring of 2022. She shares juicing recipes, tips and health benefits in a clean, simple aesthetic, attracting thousands to her online community. Her goal is to meet people where they are in their wellness journey and to create a space where a healthy lifestyle is attainable.

Jeanette currently lives in Kalamazoo, Michigan, with her husband, Jeremy. She graduated from Grand Valley State University with a bachelor's degree in marketing, and she has over six years of marketing experience in the grocery, food and beverage industry. She enjoys trying to re-create her mom's Mexican dishes, finding fun ways to stay active and trying new food experiences with friends and family. You can find more about her content and juices on her Instagram page @juicyjuicingj.

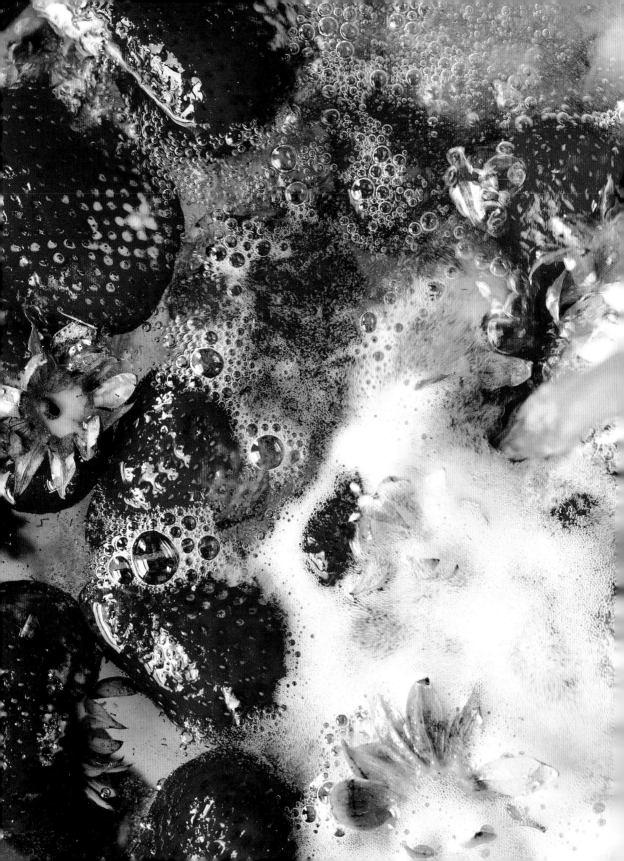

INDEX